K. E. Bergmann,
R. L. Bergmann

Health Promotion
and
Disease Prevention
in the Family

Foreword

Our health system resembles a repair service which treats illness and suffering in a gigantic economic operation. But in the case of many health problems it would seem to be much simpler to avoid them. Why do we wait and wait until the illnesses have developed? The reason is probably that we still see health as a natural resource that we can exploit to achieve our life-goals and to feel good. As long as this resource is still available we see no reason at all to spend any of our costly living time in keeping healthy.

The fact that such a large proportion of the population is prepared to ruin their health by activities such as smoking, binge drinking, drunk-driving, drug taking, physical inactivity, or gluttony, mindless of the harmful consequences such a lung cancer, injuries, diabetes, cardiovascular problems, blindness and early death, has led to many in the health system adopting a fatalistic attitude. But it would be wrong to overlook the successes of prevention. Despite increasing traffic densities, road fatalities have declined appreciably over recent decades; teeth are less affected by caries; many infectious diseases are avoided by vaccinations; improved hygiene has forced numerous (often deadly) illnesses into the background. Life expectancy, for example of the German population, has doubled within only a hundred years. And in the United States the prevalence of cigarette smoking has been reduced considerably. So it would be very wrong to say that prevention has not achieved anything.

In the field of prevention of illnesses one frequently misses (1) a scientifically-based aetiology, (2) specific goals in terms of how much of what should be achieved within what period, (3) scientifically evaluated prevention strategies, (4) customer orientation, and (5) the adaptation of the approach to the specific prevention requirement (promoting breast-feeding, for example, will require a different strategy than road accident prevention), this principle being neglected too often.

It seems to us to be particularly important to address the people who have a positive attitude to prevention. Young and expectant families are a particularly good example, because they are in a phase of reorientation. According to the results of our representative surveys they are particularly interested in maintaining the health of their children and the whole family. Since prevention must begin long before the emergence of illness, there can be no better time to start than the beginning of life – so that young and expectant families are again the ideal addressees. Young families are probably the most important and most promising target group when it comes to putting over a lifestyle which maintains health.

This book considers how to transmit ideas about maintaining health and safety to these young families. It looks at the most important concerns of prevention, and the authors analyse what should be transmitted and how the message can be got across most effectively, in a way directly relevant for the lives and lifestyles of individual people. We hope readers will find that this book contains a good mix of theoretical and practical contributions, that will not only encourage reflection about the problems discussed but will also provide practical tips for action.

We are grateful to all the contributors, many of whom initially made their expertise available to a symposium held in Berlin, while others have contributed individual chapters. I would also like to thank Henrike Bergmann-Fritsch and Richard Holmes for the editing and translating of contributions. Finally I am grateful to all those who chaired or participated in the symposium sessions and discussions, und have helped in this way to clarify that prevention really can be better than cure.

Prof. Dr. Renate L. Bergmann

Prof. Dr. Johannes Brodehl   Prof. Dr. Karl E. Bergmann

Contents

List of Contributors

Sibylle Becker, Head of the Division of Health Promotion, AOK Bundesverband, Cologne, Germany

Prof. Dr. Karl E. Bergmann, Chairman, Kaiserin Auguste Victoria (KAV) Society for Preventive Paediatrics. Speaker for Prevention, German Academy of Paediatrics. Head of the division 2.3: Health of Children and Adolescents, Prevention Concepts, Robert Koch-Institute (Federal Institute of Public Health), Berlin, Germany

Prof. Dr. Renate L. Bergmann, Chairwomen of the KAV-Institute of Preventive Paediatrics. Prof. of Pediatrics, Dept. of Obstetrics, Charité-Virchow Hospitals and Clinics, Humboldt-University, Berlin, Germany

Prof. Dr. Johannes Brodehl, Secretary General, German Academy of Paediatrics, Hannover, Germany

Prof. Dr. Sieghart Dittmann, Member of the German Advisory Committee on Immunisation, Former Chief, Communicable Disease and Immunisation Programmes, WHO Regional Office for Europe, Copenhagen, Denmark

Prof. Dr. Joachim W. Dudenhausen, Chairman, Department of Obstetrics, Charité-Virchow Hospitals and Clinics, Humboldt University, Berlin

Gerald Furian, Mag. Research Officer, Austrian Institute for Home and Leisure Safety, Vienna, Austria

Michaela Gruber, Mag., Child Safety Officer, Austrian Institute for Home and Leisure Safety, Vienna, Austria

Panagiotis Kamtsiuris, Dr. Monika Huber, Dr. Stefan Schulze, Dr. Heidrun Kahe, Uwe Schäfer Division 2.3: Health of Children and Adolescents, Prevention Concepts. Robert Koch-Institute (Federal Institute of Public Health), Berlin, Germany

Prof. Dr. Kurt Kreppner, Max Planck-Institute for Human Development, Berlin, Germany

Dr. Christiane Meyer, Dept. of Infectious Diseases Epidemiology, Robert Koch Institute, Berlin, Germany

Dr. Prümel-Philippsen, Bundesvereinigung für Gesundheit, Bonn, Germany

Dr. Gernot Rasch, Dept. of Infectious Diseases Epidemiology, Manager of the STIKO (Continuing Vaccination Committee), Robert Koch Institute, Berlin, Germany

Dr. Sabine Reiter, Dept. of Infectious Diseases Epidemiology, Robert Koch Institute, Berlin, Germany

Inke Schmidt, Speaker, Federal Working Group "Child Safety", Bonn, Germany.

PD Dr. Peter-Ernst Schnabel, Faculty of Health Sciences/Public Health, University of Bielefeld, Germany

Prof. Dr. Svante Twetman, Department of Odontology, Pedodontics, Umeå University, Umeå, Sweden

Monika Vonberg, Speaker of the Division of Education, Malteser Academy, Diözese Köln, Germany

Prof. Dr. Ulrich Wahn, Chairman, Dept. of Paediatrics, Charité Virchow Hopitals and Clinics of the Humboldt-University, Berlin, Germany

Prof. Dr. Dieter Wolke, PhD Prof. of Psychology, Unit of Peadiatric and Perinatal Epidemiology, Div. of Child Health, University of Bristol, England.

1 Health promotion and disease prevention in young families – Avoidable health problems, and expectations of young parents

Karl E. Bergmann, Renate L. Bergmann, Panagiotis Kamtsiuris, Monika Huber, Stefan Schulze, Uwe Schäfer, Heidrun Kahl

1.1 Introduction

With respect to health, mortality and longevity, the 20th century was a period of unprecedented changes: Maternal and infant mortality decreased by a factor of more than 50, the mortality of children between 1 and 15 years of age even by a factor of 65! One hundred years ago, more than 25% of the children lost their mother, and an even greater proportion of the children lost their father due to early death; orphanages were a normal part of public life. At the beginning of the 21st century orphanages have virtually disappeared. While there is still avoidable premature mortality, the interest of the public, and of health politics in death has decreased: The WHO-slogan 'add years to life' was changed to 'add life to years'. The major emphasis is now on health economics and on health related quality of life. In affluent regions, such as in the EC, USA or the Far East, medical facilities and hospitals are equipped with up-to-date technology and knowledge for the treatment of diseases and trauma, and in most of these countries, society supports and ensures medical care and protects patients from the economic risks of disease.

However, these impressive developments have not eradicated all health problems, but they have changed the focus, the concerns and the objectives in health matters, and without doubt, many preventable health problems remained: millions of children suffer injuries through accidents each year – with almost 700 children killed every year by accidents in Germany alone; children learn risky social and health behaviour early in life through family transmission that may stand in the way of a happy, healthy, and successful life and give rise to the diseases of modern civilisation, as well as developmental deficits, psychological and behavioural problems later in life. It appears that maintaining and improving the health status, and health related quality of life to meet modern expectations is even more expensive than avoiding premature death. The economic burden of less life threatening illnesses and health abnormalities is even higher than what it was when the major objective was to avoid dying. The expenses of diseases are consuming resources needed for other public and private investments for a fulfilling social and personal life.

Successful prevention has to start long before first signs of disease or abnormalities can be recognised, and in most instances this means early in life. Due to their natural helplessness, infants and children depend totally on their parents and caregivers. Most mothers and fathers are aware of their enormous responsibility. In Germany, for example, 95% of the regular paediatric check-ups are attended by the parents. However, these check-ups are confined to early signs of illness. They do not include advice about the (primary) prevention of diseases and accidents. Therefore, parents are not sufficiently prepared for their responsibility. They do not have adequate knowledge and abilities. They do not know how to promote their children's health and development. They may not be prepared to identify themselves with their role as parents. They may in many instances not be able to build up and maintain the good relationship essential for the development of healthy family structures. And finally, they may not pay sufficient attention to their own needs.

Today, almost every young person learns how to drive a car and spends plenty of time and money taking driving lessons. But no certificate is needed for the highly responsible and complicated tasks of maintaining a healthy relationship and providing adequate love and care for developing infants and children. Apart from very basic child care courses, adequate knowledge on how to raise children in a nurturing and positive environment is hardly taught anywhere. Something must be done to change this situation.

Another aspect needs to be mentioned here: While suffering is the motive for ill people to seek medical care, there is no such pressure on healthy people. Extra efforts are required to motivate them to acquire the knowledge and abilities to prevent diseases and accidents, to put their knowledge into practice and comply at least most of the time with what they have learned.

The following report introduces ideas on health promotion from early infancy on. The aim is to create a solid foundation for a long and fulfilled life for many people through prevention of diseases, injuries, and health risks. Three factors are of special importance to us: 1) a basic demand for prevention should exist; 2) only well established and proven facts should be taught; and 3) prevention programmes should take into account the needs, and the expectations of parents.

1.2   What can be prevented?

1.2.1 Health problems in infancy and childhood

Table 1.1 summarises health problems (i.e. mortality, morbidity, and risks) in infancy and childhood that are − at least in part − preventable. Three categories should be distinguished: Category [A] includes health problems scientifically proved to be preventable in experimental as well as large scale population-based studies. Category [B] comprises health problems that should be preventable according to epidemiological as well as patho-physiological knowledge, but for which no effective prevention strategies have yet been found. In this category, more population oriented research is needed to develop adequate prevention programmes. Categories [A] and [B] are not always very clearly distinguishable. Prevention options for health problems of category [C] by and large have not yet been considered.

Table 1.1: Examples of (at least partially) preventable mortality, diseases, injuries, and risks, in infancy and childhood

Category [A] Health Problems proven to be − at least in part − preventable:
- Infectious diseases preventable through vaccination
- Mortality and injuries from accidents, intoxication, foreign-body aspiration
- Sudden infant death (SIDS)
- Nutritional deficiencies (e. g. folate, vitamin D, iron, zinc, iodine, fluoride)
- Dental caries, nursing-bottle caries
- Infant diarrhoea, hypertonic dehydration
- Otitis media, diaper rash
- Insufficient physical activity
- Passive smoking and associated health problems such as respiratory diseases
- Sunburn
- Consequences of inborn errors of metabolism

Category [B] Problems (prevention conceivable, effective strategies missing):
- Premature birth
- Obesity
- Hearing loss and visual impairment
- Addiction
- Child neglect, child abuse
- Anti-social behaviour
- Learning disorders and associated problems
- Allergies
- Type I diabetes mellitus

1.2.2 Life style and prevention of diseases of modern civilisation

Life style involves learning and priming processes in early childhood and is passed on from generation to generation. We can call it cultural or family transmission. Young parents experience a period of significant insecurity and unease, in which they are very interested in reliable information, and are ready to improve their own lifestyle in support of their children's well being and perspectives of life.

Table 1.2 summarises diseases of modern civilisation that are − at least to some extent − caused by cultural and family transmission (and probably also influenced by genetic factors). In these instances, parents should be encouraged to be a good example so that their children will learn a life style that can help prevent diseases.

According to prevention options, most diseases of modern civilisation are classified as category [B] problems. More experimental and population-based research is necessary to determine the efficacy of possible prevention strategies.

A famous educator's statement "Upbringing is love and example, and not more" may appear too simple. However, it is known, that risky parental behaviour may be transmitted to the child, and should therefore be addressed in a disease prevention programme for children (Table 1.3).

Table 1.2: Diseases of modern civilisation and problems caused to some extent by early acquisition of life styles

- Adult obesity
- Type II diabetes and associated problems
- Acquired dyslipidemia
- Hypertension
- Cardiovascular diseases, myocardial infarction, Stroke
- Tooth decay, loss of teeth
- Accident morbidity and mortality
- Lung cancer, oropharyngeal tumours, bladder and gastric carcinoma
- Cervical, corporal, and breast cancer, malignant melanoma
- Arthrosis, osteoporotic bone fractures, dorsopathies
- Liver cirrhosis
- Chronic obstructive lung disease
- Suicide
- HIV-infection, AIDS
- Social deprivation, crime, drug addiction
- Contact eczema, atopy, allergy
- Depression
  Dementia

Table 1.3: Parental risk behaviour (cultural/family transmission)

- **Overweight and underweight** parents also represent a risk for the child
- **Physical activity and eating habits** are learnt by the child and are not only very important for the parents
- **Cigarette smoking** imposes an enormous health risk for parents and children, and is transmitted to the next generation with a high rate
- **Alcohol and drug abuse** are dangerous and are copied by the child
- **Risky behaviour** at work, at home, during leisure activities and in the traffic is not only dangerous but also a bad example for the children
- **A good relationship** gives children security, they copy their parents' interactive behaviour
- **Leisure time** with parents and children creates happiness and is passed on to the next generation
- **The social situation** of families can be improved: Get informed about sources of governmental and other support
- **Child abuse:** If both parents take responsibility for the protection and well-being of their child, abuse can be prevented
- If parents do not **care** enough for their **own health**, they put themselves at risk and are also a bad example

Table 1.4: Good parenting practices (GPP), selected aspects:

- The child is welcome or welcomed.
- Good parents give their child love and attention.
- Good parents try to prevent diseases, accidents and health risks.
- Good parents know their child very well and are able to satisfy his or her needs.
- They play with their child and use toys adequate for the child's developmental stage.
- They talk to their child and react to the sounds their baby makes.
- They give their child safety, knowledge, skills, and culture.
- They are reliable, understanding and consistent.
- Good parents are good partners to each other.
- They also pay regard to their own needs, and take good care of themselves.
- Family planning also respects the needs of existing children.
- Good parents make themselves and their children a happy life.
- Children can take over the life style of good parents.
- Any perfectionism is unnecessary.
- **Good parents make mistakes!**

Good parenting practices (GPP) have not been issued as rules. They may be important factors for health promotion, disease and accident prevention and for acquiring a healthy life style. Table 1.4 presents some examples.

1.3 Selected prevention issues (see also extra chapters)

1.3.1 Injuries

Accidents are the most common cause of death in children in industrialised countries. Accident mortality in children has decreased considerably in the past decades, and is now only 1/3 of the rates in 1970. Compared to other countries, Germany holds an average position in accident mortality, but ranks high in accident incidence. While excellent statistical data is available about traffic accidents, home and leisure accidents are poorly registered (Dörries et al. 1997). Traffic accident prevention largely depends on legal and technical measures related to environment and conditions as well as through traffic education starting at nursery schools and schools. Many of these measures are effective. But for accidents happening at home or during leisure activities, families are responsible. For improvements, the promising approaches are increasing product safety, making homes and environments of families and children safer, and offering anticipatory guidance.

1.3.2 Infectious diseases preventable by vaccination

In recent decades, infectious diseases have become increasingly preventable through vaccinations. But vaccination rates in Germany are still unsatisfactory. Under these circumstances, diseases preventable by vaccination such as measles or whooping cough occur much more frequently in Germany than in other countries, and it will hardly be possible to eliminate them under present conditions.

Some studies indicate that poor vaccination rates in Germany are not necessarily due to general rejection by the population, but are probably attributable to a lack of confidence among physicians [Grundhever, Stück, 1996]. However, the results of a survey we carried out in expectant and young families show that most parents are highly interested in information on vaccinations necessary for their children.

Paediatricians, on the other hand, often complain about an uncertain legal situation regarding vaccinations. The efforts required to inform parents and to obtain the legal approval of the vaccination are considered to be out of all proportion to the fee of about euro 7 per vaccination. If anything is to be improved in this matter, the structural and legal situation for the paediatricians has to be changed. Vaccinations should also become a topic of anticipatory guidance. Parents' vaccination status could be included. Since this workshop, anticipatory guidance has been tested in a controlled trial. Relatively few issues had to be addressed:

- Vaccinations are only offered for infectious diseases that can cause death and/or serious health problems.
- An independent committee newly appointed every few years by the German government evaluates the epidemiological situation with respect to the preventable infectious diseases, the vaccination status of the population, reported adverse effects of vaccinations, recent developments in the field of vaccines, especially with respect to their safety, and to vaccine combinations, the international literature for new scientific knowledge, and concerns coming from the public. The benefits and potential risks of vaccinations are compared, and vaccination schedules are reviewed.
- On the basis of the information evaluated, agreements are reached and vaccination schedules are recommended to the general population or special risk groups.
- Nearly nothing we do is completely free of risks. Serious adverse effects of vaccinations are extremely rare. Where they are reported, a government institution pays for compensation.

For more details, see extra chapter on vaccinations.

1.3.3 Nutrition related diseases in infants and children

The important issues in this area are breast feeding for a sufficient period (≥ 6 months), hygiene in the preparation of food for infants, adequate supply of micronutrients such as iodine, iron (possibly also other trace elements), vitamin K, vitamin D, fluoride, the selection of weaning foods, as well as the prevention of the "nursing bottle syndrome" and allergies (see extra chapter).

It can be assumed that about one third of all infants will suffer at least one episode of diarrhoea, and that significant proportions of infants are not supplied with adequate amounts of iron and iodine. Vitamin K deficiency occurs even under favourable conditions in developed countries, especially in breast-fed infants. All of these problems can be prevented.

1.3.4 Smoking and passive smoking in pregnancy and in families

Smoking in pregnancy leads to intrauterine growth retardation and foetal damage. Some women stop smoking during pregnancy, but restart as soon as their child is born. About half of the children in Germany have at least one smoking parent and are frequently exposed to cigarette smoke. Passive smoking is accompanied by significant health problems in children; in addition, children copy their parents' smoking habits later in life. Unfortunately, smoking is often not even addressed by obstetricians and paediatricians so that parents might get the impression that smoking does not constitute a problem at all. Prevention programmes should be designed to change the situation and to convince expectant and young parents to stop smoking, and to support them.

1.3.5 Prevention of violence against children

Article 19 of the 1989 Children's Rights Convention of the United Nations reads: "Every child is to be protected from any kind of physical and mental violence, damage, abuse, neglect, ill treatment and exploitation including sexual abuse ...".

According to police statistics from Germany, 115 000 children were injured in 1995, and 568 (349 aged 0–14 years) were killed through violent assaults. Large numbers remain undiscovered. Based on the 1989 UN definition, violence against children is probably very widespread. Risk factors for violence against children can be recognised to a certain degree, so that it is possible to help parents avoid violence, especially with regard to physical injuries and psychological problems.

1.3.6 Allergy prevention (see extra chapter)

Allergies are not only very common, but also as a public health problem are gaining increasing attention and public concern in developed countries. Allergy prevention should be an important issue. According to several controlled intervention and observational studies, (early) exposure to allergens and harmful substances such as car exhaust, cigarette smoke, or ozone should be avoided. It is very likely that many opinions on allergies will change in the near future, making allergies a typical category B problem.

1.3.7 Nutritional deficits in pregnancy

The importance of pre- and postnatal nutrition for mother and child may be under-estimated. Not all pregnant women in Germany receive iodine and (early) folic acid supplements; iron deficiency is not uncommon in later pregnancy. Weight gains during pregnancy are not sufficiently corrected after birth, so that obesity is very wide-spread in the German female population. Nutrition deficits in part also account for prematurity. Prevention programmes with the aim of improving health in parents and children are not possible without good nutrition for pregnant women (Berg-mann et al., Deutsches Ärzteblatt 1997).

1.3.8 Prevention of damage caused by alcohol

In Germany, 170 000 to 340 000 women aged 20−49 years are thought to suffer from alcoholism. It is well-established that alcohol consumption during pregnancy can cause severe foetal damage. Due to widespread alcohol abuse, foetal alcohol syndrome is a significant health risk in the German population. Following prevention options have been proposed:

- Better information of the population − especially of young and pregnant women − on the dangers of alcohol consumption during pregnancy.
- Improvement of maternity guidelines: pregnant women must be informed about the dangers of alcohol consumption during pregnancy.
- Women at risk should receive efficient education as early as possible.
- Organisation of specialised health centres for women with addiction problems.
- Hospitalisation of pregnant women addicted to alcohol in special wards.
- Establishment of structures for the attendance of pregnant women addicted to alcohol. The public health service (PHS) in Germany is entitled to follow up on families and persons not using the health system, to offer advice and help to such families. The PHS should be educated, equipped and structured to help women addicted or prone to addiction.

1.3.9 Prevention of premature birth

In Germany, the proportion of infants born before 37 weeks of gestation and/or with birth weights under 2 500 g has increased during recent years to about 5 to 8 % of all live births. Prematurity rates vary significantly between regions and countries. Prematurity is one of the main reasons for infant mortality and severe permanent physical and mental impairments. In Germany the total expenses for the treatment of very low birth weight (VLBW) infants were estimated to be Euro 200 million in 1994.

The aetiology of premature birth is still not fully understood. Numerous risk factors have been identified, some of which are amenable to primary preventive measures.

They include infections, smoking, hypertension low body weight and nutritional deficiencies. Premature birth is a preventable health problem of category B. Apart from further etiological research on premature birth, prevention studies may be carried out to evaluate efficacy, acceptance, as well as cost effectiveness of measures derived from current knowledge.

1.3.10 Gestational diabetes

Gestational diabetes may cause foetal damage. Previously, the prevalence of gestational diabetes was underestimated. In Germany, about 8 to 14% of pregnant women are likely to have gestational diabetes. In many cases, this problem is being diagnosed. As far as the mother is concerned, gestational diabetes is a matter of early identification of the disease, and consequently a problem of secondary prevention. For the child, gestational diabetes is a true health risk requiring primary prevention measures. An improvement of screening strategies benefits both mother and child. If maternal diabetes is well stabilised during pregnancy, malformations, growth disorders, and birth complications can (at least in part) be prevented. Generally, gestational diabetes can be viewed as a category B problem. Large scale prevention measures should be preceded and accompanied by well evaluated model projects.

1.3.11 Early prevention of health risks in later life

Preventive measures only concentrating on the specific health problems of childhood are not sufficient. If civilisation diseases, accident injuries and mortality, psychological disorders, addiction, and anti-social behaviour are to be prevented, a healthy lifestyle has to be established early in life. This requires people to be able to take responsibility for their own life and health. These abilities are not only associated with the social and economic situation of the family, but also relate to the ability of the parents to promote the child's independence, to their competence in health matters, and the quality of their relationship.

One very important factor is the parents' knowledge of the natural course of their child's development, abilities, immaturity and of the child's needs (Largo, 1995) as well as of setting limits. According to Brazelton (1995), children develop "discontinuously". Periods of intensive development also exert a strong influence on the child's environment; Brazelton refers to them as "touch-points".

A prevention programme with the aim of achieving long-term health must be designed according to (1) the development of the child; (2) the achievements, pleasures and problems associated with the child's development; (3) the social and economic situation of the family, as well as their habits and way of life; and (4) adaptation processes of parents and children to ever changing situations. Consultation has to take into account the knowledge, the abilities, the situation, and the values of individual families and their environment (Contextual Pediatrics, Green, 1995).

In this sense, the foundations for life style, competence, independence and the ability to take responsibility for oneself are laid very early in life. Early prevention of civilization diseases, accident risks, and behavioural disorders are issues of the category B.

1.4   Target Groups, demand and options

1.4.1 Institutional prevention programmes for children and adolescents

Children and adolescents have long been a target group for prevention. Schools, nursery schools etc. are often being utilised for preventive measures. Extensive strategies and programmes were designed for these purposes by institutions such as the German Federal Centre for Health Education (Bundeszentrale für Gesundheitliche Aufklärung).

However, health and healthy lifestyles are not the focus of interest for young people. They would rather explore many areas of life utilising or even consuming their own health resources − with an almost limitless self-confidence. Frequently, it is socially unacceptable for adolescents to show healthy behaviour too openly. Therefore, health education for young people has to make use of strong incentives, motivation, and social support. Even then, it is not too often successful.

1.4.2 Families as target groups for preventive measures

In this respect, expectant and young families have a completely different attitude. Feeling responsible for their own children and concerned with their health and life perspectives, parents show a natural interest for information and are open for health issues. They want to learn about their child's developmental milestones, how to treat and educate their children, about life style and maintaining a healthy relationship. Young parents can display healthy behaviour everywhere. Obviously, there is a legitimate demand for competent information and counselling. But is adequate education and information available in Germany?

Early diagnosis of diseases is necessary, but not sufficient.
Pediatric prevention according to the German Social Law Code (Section 26 SGB V) is basically restricted to early diagnosis of diseases and disorders requiring medical treatment. As a programme of secondary prevention, it is carried out by paediatricians or general practitioners, and is utilised by more than 90% of German families, especially in the first year of life. But primary prevention of diseases, as well as physical, mental, and social disorders, injuries, and risky habits leading to diseases of modern civilisation later in life must begin before early symptoms and problems occur.

This type of primary prevention was previously offered by public health service clinics. Paediatric and general practitioners are focused on curative medicine. They are paid for treatment and early diagnosis, but not for primary prevention. Hardly any of them are trained in the area of health promotion, primary prevention of diseases and of injuries, and therefore rarely offer information on such topics.

Much of health related lifestyle is acquired early in childhood and passed on from generation to generation. We call it the cultural or family transmission. Expectant and young parents experience a period of significant insecurity, in which they are very interested in information, and are ready to improve their lifestyle for the sake of their children's well-being.

But since most of the mother and child units of the public health service have been closed, parents are not informed about prevention, and they do not learn anything about healthy lifestyles, their child's normal development, or about bringing up their child.

Usually disease prevention is based largely on epidemiological and patho-physiological knowledge. If recommendations and preventive measures are ineffective, or not well accepted, we probably did not know about the needs and request of our target groups. Maybe we forgot to ask the people we were addressing whether they want the information at all, what their expectations and interests are, and how and by whom advice should be given.

1.4.3 Needs and demand of expectant and young parents

In order to avoid this widespread mistake, we carried out a representative study among women in 109 obstetric and maternity wards (10% of those in Germany) in 1997. Of 7825 questionnaires distributed, 5900 (75.4%) were filled in completely; 12.7% of the questionnaires were answered by pregnant women or expectant couples, 48.1% had at least one child already.

1.4.3.1 Request for intensive anticipatory guidance

73.4% of expectant or young parents were convinced that intensive anticipatory guidance for themselves and their children was necessary. 24.7% of the parents wanted advice only on specific request, and 1.9% of all did not find any anticipatory guidance necessary (fig. 1.1).

According to 95% of the parents, prevention should be offered in paediatric practices. Nursery schools, maternity wards, and health insurance offices were seen as optional locations for preventive health education by 27 to 52% of the parents. Public health stations (18%), obstetric practice (10%) were of less interest. According to this survey, all other institutions appear unimportant to most of the participants (fig. 1.2).

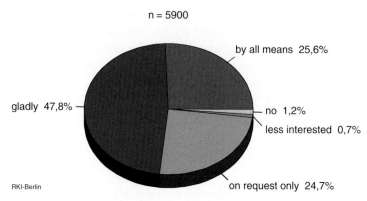

Fig. 1.1: Do you want to be advised about the prevention of diseases and injuries, and about understanding and educating your child?

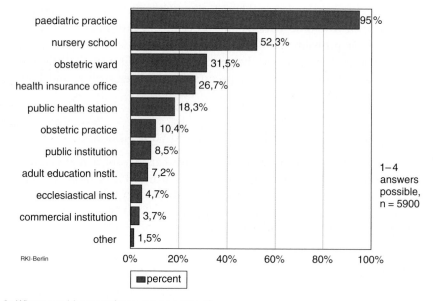

Fig. 1.2: Where would you prefer to get counseled?

89.8% of the parents would like advice on health promotion and disease prevention to be offered by a physician, 68.8% would accept advice from a midwife, and 60.3% also from a paediatric nurse. All other professions are considerably less accepted (fig. 1.3). The high acceptance of doctors, midwives, and paediatric nurses should be utilised for prevention programmes. These expectations and statements of confidence call for the education of these professions: Doctors, midwives, and nurses should be specifically trained to provide anticipatory guidance. Of course, the accep-

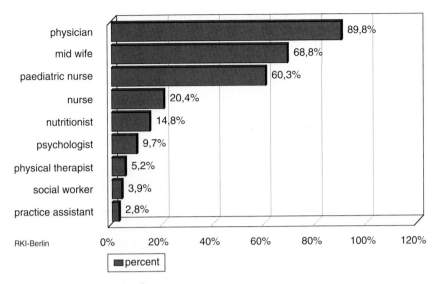

Fig. 1.3: Who could be your advisor?

tance of these professions is also related to the fact that they are familiar to many parents.

Over 85% of the parents wished for personal consultations. Information brochures, parent groups, books, information series for parents, telecasts, pamphlets and magazines were in the medium range with 26 to 36%. Videos and multimedia offers, especially via internet were of lesser interest (fig. 1.4).

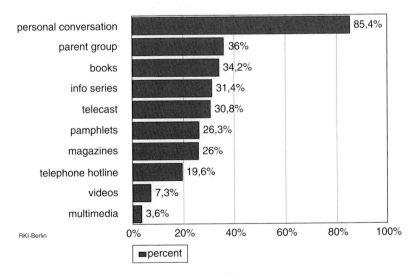

Fig. 1.4: Which type of communication would you prefer?

1.4.4 Issues of special interest from the mothers' point of view

During pregnancy, parents are not only interested in the intrauterine development of the child (96 %) and for the preparation of birth (95 %), but naturally also for issues relevant after birth such as breast feeding and nutrition (93 %) as well as the new born infant (88 %). Even information on disease prevention, healthy life style, and good parenthood are interesting for large proportions of the parents (fig. 1.5).

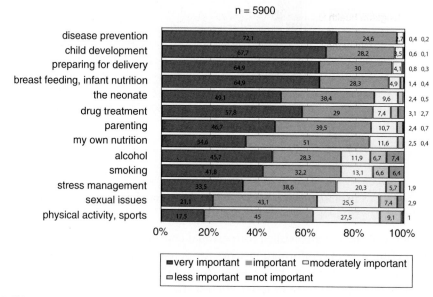

Fig. 1.5: What would you like to be advised about during pregnancy?

During the child's first years, 96 % of the parents are most interested in vaccinations and the management of diseases. But health preservation, good nutrition, and the better understanding of the needs of the child are highly interesting for most parents. How to deal with crying babies and baby and child care also get many points. The questions, "what can I do to make my child live long", and, "how can I prevent accidents" are still interesting for more than half of the parents. If the possible answers "very interesting" and "moderately interesting" are added up, there is a desire for counselling for all issues from more than 60 % of parents.

However, the mothers' own well-being is considered to be less important (fig. 1.6).

1.4.5 Differences between groups, Cluster analysis

Are expectations similar in all socio-demographic groups? This aspect was analysed in two steps: (1) A factorial analysis of the questions showed that 75 % of them could be assigned to four factors, Fig. 1.7.:

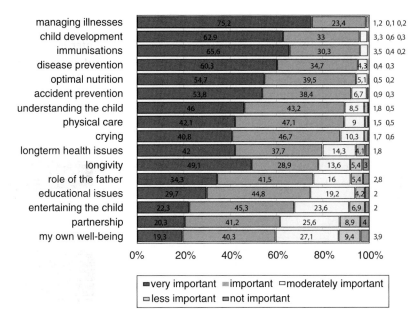

Fig. 1.6: What would you want to be advised about during the first years of your child?

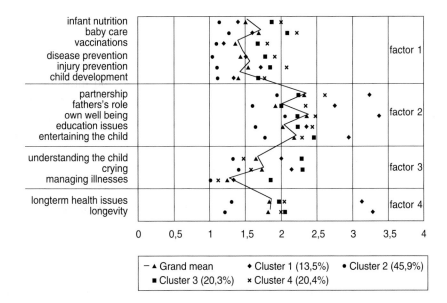

Fig. 1.7: What would you want to be advised about during the first years of your child?

The factors could be described and termed as follows:

Factor 1: main prevention issues
Factor 2: interaction in the family
Factor 3: caring
Factor 4: concerned about the future.

(2) Fig. 1.8 shows how the cluster analysis assigned clusters and their components, the answers, to the factors. The clusters have typical patterns with respect to the weight every of the factors is given in each of the clusters of respondent parents.

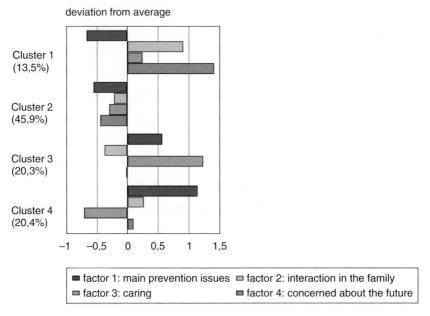

Fig. 1.8: Cluster analysis

All clusters contain some of everything. However, if we look at them more closely, we see the following picture (statistically significant deviations from average):

Mothers in cluster 1:

Above average: Have/expect first child, have polytechnic degree.
Below average: From West Germany, incomplete education.

Mothers in cluster 2:

Above average: Have/expect first child, incomplete education, age under 25 years, live in cities of more than 50 000 and less than 1 million. Below average: Age between 26 and 40, polytechnic and university degree.

Mothers in cluster 3:

Above average: Have children already, are between 26 and 40 years of age, from West Germany. Below average: Under 25 years of age, in cities of 1 million or more. No influence of educational level.

Mothers in cluster 4:

Above average: university degree; marginal significance: city of ≥ 1 million, age ≥ 41 years, first child, West Germany (incl. West Berlin).
Below average: From communities of $\leq 500\,000$. Marginal: age under 25.

1.4.6 Organization aspects of anticipatory guidance

During pregnancy, 55% of parents would like to have one single consultation for all issues, but 45% would also agree to come two or three times. No strong preference for a certain period of gestation. However, the period between the 4th and 6th month of pregnancy seems to be favoured by more than half (fig. 1.9).

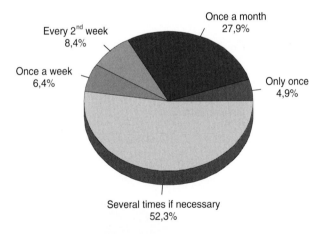

Fig. 1.9: How often would you come for advice?

The request for information appears to be much greater during the child's first year: only 5% of parents consider one single consultation to be sufficient. Most parents would like to have their consultation together with the regular paediatric check-up, equivalent to 5 to 6 appointments during the first year of life. Mothers also think that much information is needed immediately after birth. Counselling at the start of nursery school is regarded less important. Asked in a different way their answers are as follows: 28% would come at least once a month, 15% even more often 52% several times but only, if necessary.

About half of the parents would agree to a duration of 30–60 minutes; without their children, 32% of parents would even like to have 90 minutes consultation (fig. 1.10)

About half of the parents would like to come in the evening, one quarter prefers afternoon and one quarter prefers morning hours.

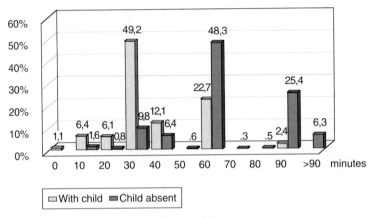

Fig. 1.10: Acceptable duration of one session

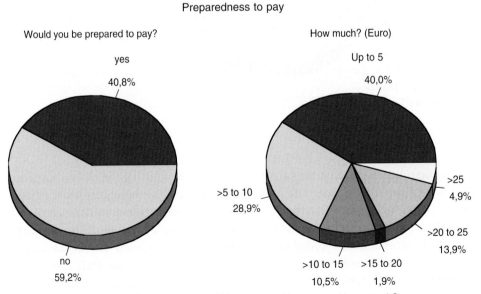

Fig. 1.11 What proportion of the parents would be prepared to pay, and how much?

1.5 Prevention and Economy

Disease prevention in the family should not only be focused on early identification of diseases, but also have the aim of risk reduction and prevention of category A problems. If anticipatory guidance of young families could be added to the pediatric prevention programme in Germany, disease prevention would be more efficient, and family health could be improved significantly. The introduction of prevention programmes of this type in other places was not only medically but also economically successful. Miller and Galbraith (1995) showed a cost-benefit ratio of 1/13 for "The Injury Prevention Programme" of the American Academy of Pediatrics for children aged 0−4 years. Similar positive results were also achieved in the national anti-smoking-programme for pregnant women in the United States that was economically evaluated by Marks et al. (1990). The authors found a cost-benefit ratio of 1/6.58.

However, primary prevention programmes are economically justified (increasing efficiency) only by truly efficient achievements. For this reason, one of the main tasks must be economic evaluations of preventive measures, including correlation analysis and evaluation of outcomes, processes and structures, as well as an efficiency assessment through cost-benefit analysis.

1.6 Summary and conclusions

Mortality, premature death, longevity, and morbidity have improved dramatically during the 20th century, resulting in a life expectancy unprecedented in the history of mankind. Hygiene, nutrition and economic development, medical care, as well as vaccination programmes and prevention measures for malnutrition, rickets and dental caries have greatly contributed to the health of pregnant women, infants and children. Thereby, the understanding of health and disease have changed with the interest in mortality decreasing for an increasing attention for health related quality of life as well as economic aspects of health care.

These are the reasons for new concerns with respect to health problems, health risks and accidents. Many of them appear to be preventable. Getting people to avoid such problems requires completely different approaches than in the treatment of diseases.

First of all, avoidable health problems should be identified and as a next step, intervention strategies can be conceptualised and implemented. This includes (1) Deciding what can be done e. g. wearing helmets, seat belts, using fluoride for caries prevention, decreasing fat intake, increasing physical activity etc., (2) Identifying the parts of the population to be addressed, (3) Finding out how they can be approached efficiently, (4) Developing a vision to be shared at community level, objectives and programmes, (5) Obtaining funds, (6) Implementing the programmes, and finally (7) Evaluating the processes and structures as well as monitoring the outcomes.

This chapter starts out presenting health problems in early childhood amenable to prevention. But its major contribution is the analysis of the demand on the part of the population to be addressed, i. e. expecting and young parents:

Demand for prevention:
Results of a representative survey among 5900 expectant and young parents in Germany show that the majority of them have a great demand for competent anticipatory guidance. The parents apparently trust their physicians, midwifes or paediatric nurses and would accept advice from them in an interactive, personal way about quite a broad spectrum of topics. Prenatally, one appointment appears to be sufficient to the majority of them, but during the first year of life, they prefer to see their advisor more frequently. Age of the mother, her educational status, existing experience with own children, diseases in the family, or the community size have an influence on the preferences, but by and large, the major topics rank high in most of them. If programmes have to be developed for larger areas, the results of our cluster analysis should be taken into account. About 40 % of the parents were prepared to pay for a programme.

Outlook:
Primary prevention in expectant and young families is likely to make itself independent eventually. Because most parents are not able to pay for prevention, and since it is very likely that good information and health education will reduce morbidity, mortality, and health expenses, it seems justified to include this type of prevention in the payment scheme of health insurances.

Prevention counsellors should get involved in continuing education, quality control should be established. For this reason the Kaiserin Auguste Viktoria Society will launch an education programme for paediatricians, obstetricians as well as other professions dealing with prevention issues. The expectations of young families regarding qualified anticipatory guidance will have a great impact on obstetrics and paediatrics: in future, prevention will be of high importance in these fields.

1.7 References

In cooperation with the Kaiserin Auguste Viktoria Institute, the Robert Koch Institute has worked out a report on prevention in the family for the German Ministry of Health which also includes a review of more than 1 000 publications. The report was financially supported by the German Ministry of Health (BMG).

1.8 Discussion

Prof. Brodehl (Chair):
In my opinion, one of the main questions is whether you can generalise your data. I think we need to know how you did this study: Did you use questionnaires, or

were the participants interviewed? How did you plan the evaluation of the data of over 5 000 participants? Could you tell us a little bit more about the methodology of this study?

Prof. Bergmann:
In Germany, we have about 1 100 maternity wards. And we drew a 10% random sample of those wards, weighted for the number of deliveries per year. Then we selected a four-week-interval and included every consecutive delivery in this hospital from mothers who were able to understand German – this was the only condition. We had many foreign mothers in this study as well, but only foreign mothers who were able to understand and answer our questions. And it was strictly consecutive, so there was no chance for the delivery wards to select any mothers for sympathy or preparedness to answer or for any other reasons. It was strictly consecutive. We distributed 7 825 questionnaires, and we had a number of people in our institute who stayed in touch with the representatives of all of the 109 maternity wards every day. The feedback was very good: 5 900 completed questionnaires (a little over 75%) were returned in time; in the remaining 25% the parents were not reluctant to answer, but rather, they were not returned in time or their distribution had not worked as well in some hospitals. For these reasons, we are convinced that our data represent the German population of expecting and young mothers of Germany, at the end of 1997.

Prof. Brodehl (Chair):
Because you have locations with few inhabitants, you must have included the country-side also. [Prof. Bergmann: Yes, we did] How did you distribute the questionnaires in Germany, I mean, it must have been a big task.

Prof. Bergmann:
Yes. A German-wide representative study. So maybe I should tell you how we did it: we drew a 10-percent sample of the 1 102 maternity wards, with some over-sampling, actually we drew a sample of 123 maternity wards. Some of the maternity wards did not exist any more, so some – I think it was five – had to be substituted by another nearby maternity ward. Finally, of the 123 maternity wards 109 co-operated. I personally talked to each of the heads of the maternity wards first, got his agreement to participate, and then sent him the written material, and with the written material we came to a decision whether the maternity ward would participate or not. The head of the department nominated a person responsible in his maternity ward to distribute the questionnaires. Every completed questionnaire was paid with DM 4 (about euro 2). I think it worked out nicely; with surveys based on questionnaires you very rarely have a 75-percent participation.

Prof. Brodehl (Chair):
Yes, I thank you very much for these details. Prof. Tietze, please!

Prof. Tietze, Berlin:
Wolfgang Tietze, Centre for Early Childhood Education, Free University. I have a question in regard to the methodology. What we know from survey research is that the context in which questions are asked may influence the responses. And so I wonder if the results would be pretty much the same if you had not asked people in the context of maternity wards but let's say in a different context. And I think, I ask this question because what the results show is that mothers mainly address the medical advisory system. And I wonder if this response pattern is influenced by the fact that they were asked in a medical context. So let us assume: you would have a different sample when mothers are at home and they are in their neighbourhood context. Also their social network, their network consisting of Church organisations or the like, so I wonder if you would get different results. And I think the question is not just a theoretical one, but it has practical implications because what I understand is: such a study, the results, could be a basis to draw conclusions: how to set up an advisory system, and if the responses are very much biased in regard to the medical system, maybe we are in danger of drawing biased conclusions.

Prof. Bergmann:
Thank you very much, Prof. Tietze. I think you are right. You can conduct quite different surveys. The important point is: we addressed parents during a period of great change and concern. Your horizon is in pre-school education, and the type of concern and expectations in pre-school children may be completely different. So not only the setting plays a role, but also the period during which you address the people. And actually our major interest was in this − I would call it − pre-institutional period of life. This is a period of life where you have difficulties to find parents to ask any questions! So if I go to a kindergarten, I can distribute a questionnaire, but how do you get to parents who have just delivered their children. Certainly, they have their recent experience, but also if you look at the type of answers − for example I would have expected that in the first place they would tell that their obstetrician would be the number-one person they would expect something from. But they expect the information from the paediatrician, despite I asked them in the delivery ward. So I think there is a mixture of influences, and we would be ill-advised if we would draw too wide-ranging conclusions. The fact that I co-operate with you, and the fact that I hopefully will have you here as one of our chairmen, shows that we do not draw these wide-ranging conclusions. We find it very helpful to have this information. Nothing comparable was available before. We need much additional information beyond this. But this what we have now.

Prof. Brodehl (Chair):
There is another question:

Prof. Dittmann:
Sieghard Dittmann, Berlin. It is the same line as Prof. Tietze. I think the results are very interesting, and particularly that you found that the doctor, the paediatrician,

is still one of the key partners. But I have also some doubts, especially when we see what role was given in this survey to the media. Because we know that particularly the media can play a very important role, both in providing good issues and bad issues, particularly bad issues. And I could give a lot of examples: we have the press, but I do not want to accuse the press − let us say: the badly advised press very quickly destroyed big programmes. So it destroyed diphtheria vaccination in Russia, and so on and so on. So I think, nevertheless I do not want to accuse you of being old-fashioned. But we should not underestimate the role of the media, and that is clearly one of the main issues in future to have very good and close co-operation with the media.

Prof. Brodehl (Chair):
Thank you. Multi-media, was only what you meant,

Prof. Bergmann:
The main point, yes. However, we included some answers of the parents with respect to their utilisation of TV and their satisfaction with it. We ourselves are not in any way against public media.

Prof. Brodehl (Chair):
yes, but only the internet was criticised, and the print media had 30 percent or so.

Prof. Bergmann:
Right.

Prof. Brodehl (Chair):
You refer to multi-media, do you?

Prof. Bergmann:
Yes that is true. Well, I do not say that I do not find the media important. We asked the parents: "would you expect something good from the media". And apparently the parents are quite critical, they are more critical than we believe. But also I can confirm your observation from e. g. the prevention of dental caries by fluoride, it was a big television show in Germany that destroyed the fluoride prophylaxis [Prof. Brodehl: (1985)] of dental caries in I think 1986 or so, and it took years to pick up and get back to a good compliance. So you are absolutely right; I'm not for disregarding the media, I asked the parents what they think they want to have.

NN:
It is a question of how you formulate your questions.

Prof. Bergmann:
Yes.

Prof. Brodehl (Chair):
That is right. Yes.

NN:
Not satisfied!

Prof. Bergmann:
Okay. The multi-media were one of several items of the question: "where would you want to get your advice from? But there are media as you said that are accepted by the people we asked, like books, that are media, [Prof. Brodehl: Books are media, also.] and they have a high rank as compared to multi-media.

Prof. Brodehl (Chair):
Any more questions? Professor Helge please

Prof. Helge:
Hans Helge, Berlin. I wonder how you made the categories of your clustering. I do not understand how this came about, but I think they are not separate, they are really interrelated, the four clusters which you showed us. And you cannot say, if you belong to one cluster you do not belong to the other one. And the clustering, to me, is a new way of dividing results, but I want to know how the clustering was done, is it something which is established with epidemiologists to have these four groups, or is this just by your own choice that by clustering you selected these four groups?

Prof. Bergmann:
In cluster analysis, an automated statistical procedure tests whether the data is homogenously distributed or whether there is any non-homogenous clustering. In the present case, it was a two step procedure: in the first step, by a factorial analysis it was tested, whether any of our questions can be grouped because the answers tend into similar directions. And we found four types of questions. It could have been three, or five, or six, but four groups explain about 75-percent of the variance. In the second step, we tested to what extent the persons answering can be assigned to the types of questions. It is an automated methodology. However, the terms used for the groups of questions and for clusters of persons were assigned by us.

Prof. Helge:
And the overlap?

Prof. Bergmann:
There is a wide overlap: the mothers who are less likely to belong to a cluster are certainly not eliminated completely from that cluster, e. g. they are not completely disinterested in the matter characterised by the type of questions. They just tend to

be less interested, and this tendency may be significant or not significant. By and large we have to say that the majority of mothers are very much interested in getting advised. But if they are very young, they apparently are somewhat less interested. And if they are from a big city, they'll belong less to cluster no. 3 and so on. So it is only a matter of probability. And it is not categorial. There is certainly overlap in the persons.

Prof. Brodehl (Chair):
Did you look for the number of children the parents had?

Prof. Bergmann:
Yes, we did.

Prof. Brodehl (Chair):
Do mothers, or fathers also, or families who have only one child care more or less about the future?

Prof. Bergmann:
Yes, that is a good question: if they have children already they tend to belong more to cluster no. 1, which is family- and future-orientation. And this is also significant. We also analysed this for the number of children, and actually into several directions. I just showed you a couple of the highlights.

Prof. Brodehl (Chair):
Thank you. Yes, please, go ahead.

Dr. Ropers:
Gwendolin Ropers is my name; associate to the Robert Koch Institute; I have a question about the fourth cluster, and you didn't tell us about the features of the fourth cluster, and can you tell us something about those people?

Prof. Bergmann:
Thank you for your question, Dr. Ropers. Actually it is a rather complex pattern, very time consuming to explain. Therefore, I would prefer not to discuss it here. But I have the results here on paper, it is about ten pages to go through. I can give it to anyone specifically interested in cluster four

Prof. Brodehl (Chair):
There is another question, please

Prof. Wolke:
Dieter Wolke from the University of Hertfordshire in England. I mean I'm not that concerned about that a lot of parents said that they go to a paediatrician, because in these questionnaires they usually answer: what they know, they will be going to.

The danger is to draw the conclusion that only paediatricians can deliver this. But it may be the point of contact where a delivery system works with, like via health nurses, health visitors, or any other system which is implemented. In Germany more than ninety percent of the women will habitually go to the paediatrician, and they have done that before. This will differ between health care systems. And the second thing which we have alluded to is the inverse health service delivery system. Those people who need it least use it most. And those who need it most use it least. Presumably that is the group more focus should be placed on, and perhaps more in-depth analysis.

Prof. Bergmann:
Yes.

Prof. Brodehl (Chair):
Thank you.

Prof. Bergmann:
Thank you very much, this would be one of our conclusions.

Prof. Brodehl (Chair):
We left some important point out of the discussion so far: the only practicing paedi-atrician I personally know in this room is Dr. Schmetz, and he should say something really, maybe later on, because there is a main focus: how can paediatricians meet the demand? Would you be prepared to react to this very important question? Dr. Schmetz, please:

Dr. Schmetz:
I would like to comment on that as this is also one of our concerns, but it concerns not only the paediatrician, but also the midwife and the paediatric nurse, who are also in the focus of the parents, (they) would want to accept their advice, and from practical observations we know that young parents rely very much on the advice of midwives! And midwives distribute in Germany quite peculiar information to par-ents, and we do have problems with the midwife. So we need to educate paediatrici-ans and every type of profession, who then distributes the knowledge to parents. None of them has it, including educators.

Prof. Brodehl (Chair):
Professor Bergmann, thank you very much, for the stimulating start to this work-shop.

2 Quality of relationship, sensitivity for developmental changes, and transition competence

– Three components for establishing good partnerships among all family members –

Kurt Kreppner

2.1 Abstract

The transmission of knowledge about family health should be based on three main components: Relationship maintenance, development sensitivity, and transition competence. These three aspects describe internal characteristics of a family's ability to support or to impede a child's individual developmental pathway; they also provide a more general framework for the parents' task to raise children.

These components constitute the foundation for mastering normative crises in parent-infant and parent-parent relationships: First, the objective of establishing and maintaining the parent-child relationship within the family after the child's arrival. Second, associated with this is the reorganisation of the marital relationship. Third, the objective of reacting sensitively to the infant's developmental changes and adapting to the growing needs and skills of the child; and third, the objective of dealing competently with family transitions.

The concept of the family as a developing unit which has to master critical transitions is illustrated by empirical data from two different periods, early childhood and adolescence. The ability to keep continuity and change in balance when reorganising relationships within a family during transition periods appears to be an essential ingredient for family functioning.

2.2 Introduction

The task of communicating knowledge, skills, and health behaviour can be accomplished in various ways. It not only depends on which information is delivered, but also on how information is being received and understood. If a young family is addressed, parents are still in a transition period from being partners of the same generation to become intergenerative partners as parents. Apart from many facts and details about a developing child, there are some fundamental issues which deserve the young parents' specific attention. The idea that knowledge on family health and child development as well as the ability to handle children can easily be taught to parents by simply transmitting facts, rules, and recipes may seem idealistic. Dealing with children has always had an additional implication: the responsibility of the present generation for the next generation. There is a long tradition in the task of instructing young parents, because at most historical times, children were educated to build a better future. In 1531, Luis Vives, a Spanish humanist and friend of Erasmus, for example, gave the following instructions to mothers on the education of their daughters (1531/1912, pp. 124/125):

> "For the babe first heareth her mother and first beginneth to inform her speech after hers. For that age can do nothing itself, but counterfeit and follow others, and is cunning in this thing only. She taketh her first conditions and information of mind by such as she heareth or seeth by her mother. Therefore, it lieth more in the mother than men when to make the conditions of the children. Let her give her diligence, at least wise because of her children, that she use no rude and blunt speech lest that manner of speaking take such root in the tender mindes of the children, and so grow and increase together with their age, that they cannot forget it. Children will learn no speach better, nor more plainly express, than they wil their mother's. ... They inquire everything to her; whatsoever she answereth, they believe and regard, and take it even for the Gospel. Oh mothers, what an occasion for you unto your children, to make them whether you will, good or bad!"

The German evolutionist Ernst Haeckel believed that during the child's development the course of evolution of the human species is replicated and therefore education is not very relevant during infancy and childhood. Psychologists like Stanley Hall developed educational programmes for adolescents to push their development beyond the natural abilities evolution had provided. Similar to the ideas of early humanism, Hall believed that by intervention during adolescence a new and enlightened generation could be created.

In the discourse about the optimisation of knowledge and moral in the next generation, one question has always been asked: What is the most appropriate context within which to foster good upbringing. As an early answer to this question, for example, Vives in 1531 proposed that mothers and even nurses should be taught in their native languages, not in Latin, in order to guarantee that they can give good education to their children.

2.3   A broader perspective for health promotion: Relationship, family development, and transitions

2.3.1 The family as the child's proximal context

If we assume that the most relevant context for infants and children are the parents, what should we communicate to young parents in order to promote well-being and health in families? Of course, all of the following is important and should be well known by parents: Facts about how a child grows up, facts about body changes, perceptual and mental abilities, locomotion, ideas about how to arrange the room in which the baby lives, information about what kind of food is appropriate at what age or how to prevent sicknesses. At the same time, however, a broader perspective could be conveyed with regard to the general concept of health in young families.

Young parents with a first child are still living in a period of transition between two major stages in their own development. They have successfully established a partner relationship and are just trying to accomplish their next developmental task, that is, to initiate and maintain an intergenerational relationship. The child grows up in the young family consisting of three dyadic relationships: Mother-father, mother-child, and father-child. Each of these dyads needs specific attention and care as the child, as the new family member, is a still largely unknown being which has to be integrated, and the parental dyad opens new perspectives on the partner as a parent on the one hand, and generates new tasks such as balancing the responsibilities for the offspring on the other. The new family member, the infant, is not a passive creature just formed by the relational context of the family. Instead, the infant is an active participant in the family relationships right from the beginning. Research over the past 25 years has amply shown the richness of babies' activities to participate in the formation of the relationship with the primary caregivers, it has also provided us with much evidence that the quality of relationship between primary caregiver and infant is essential for the child's possibilities to develop his or her abilities and skills. We have learned, for example, from a number of experiments with infants between 3 and 8 months of age that these young family members actively try to keep an interaction with the mother going if she suddenly stops exhibiting facial expressions, if her face "freezes" (still face experiments, Tronick, 1989; Tronick and Cohn, 1989). Infants begin to produce various kinds of expressions to stimulate the partner to new reactions. Other experiments have shown that babies take the mother's facial expression and gestures as signals directing their behaviour in uncertain situations for example, when they have to cross a "visual cliff" (Source, Emde, Campos, and Klinnert, 1985). At the cliff's edge children usually stop crawling and look at their mother's face. When mothers, standing at the other side of the cliff, signal danger and fear by facial expression, children do not continue to crawl onto the glass. However, when mothers encourage their children by exhibiting positive emotion and encouragement, babies cross over. About 8 months, children begin to check a parent's expression when they throw around objects or disobey rules in order to learn how far they can go (Trevarten & Hubley, 1978).

The proximal context for the infant is the family and its relational network with its particular structure and quality. Although we have seen the infant as an active participant, one has to bear in mind that the child grows up within the limits of a specific relationship with the primary caregiver, that is, with a certain standard of quality in this relationships. The child's context is also constituted by the relationship between the parents, which serves as a relevant model for the management of conflicts and the adaptation to the mutual needs of the partner. The quality of relation-

ship creates basic conditions for the possibility to communicate, correct misunderstandings, or to negotiate needs and exchange emotions (Gottman, Fainsilber-
Katz, & Hover, 1996).

2.3.2 The family context as a developing unit

During the first years with their child, the parents are confronted with rapid and
dramatic changes. Parents and child run through phases of mutual adaptation during the offspring's various developmental stages. This family-oriented view of the
interplay between parents and children during the entire life span is manifest in the
concept of family development, created by family sociologists (Duvall, 1977; Aldous,
1978). It tries to take into account the dynamic aspect of changes in the family
and to analysis crises in family interaction from the perspective of mastering family
developmental tasks, which are linked to the child's individual development, and
parents' ability, and sensitivity to adequately adapt to it. Developmental progress is
believed to be associated with all family members' well-being. This perspective on
the child's development within the context of the family broadens the possibilities to
analyse crises during the process of mutual adaptation.

2.4 Factors that contribute to coping with transitions in the family

Perhaps there is a kind of historic parallel between today's activities to convey
knowledge about family health and the birth of the concept of family development.
In 1943, after a dramatic increase in soldiers' divorces, the US army demanded that
the government develop courses to teach young couples how to live together in a
family. The situation of high rates of separation in army families had developed
during the war. Young couples married when the man was drafted to the army. He
had to go to war and came back only on short leaves. When the wife was with a
child, mutual misunderstandings and wrong interpretations of the other's intentions
increased and often ended in divorce. After the war, when soldiers came back and
stayed at home, the divorce rate grew even higher. In order to give advice to young
couples on how to organise the household to meet the needs of parents as partners
as well as the needs of the developing children, family sociologists linked Havighurst's (1948) concept of developmental tasks to the life-cycle concept. This extended
the concept of the actively developing child into a life-span development and elaborated the idea to control and sometimes push individual development by giving
advice to parents on the other hand. Evelyn Duvall and Reuben Hill published a
book entitled "When you marry" in 1945 with very practical hints about how to
avoid crises in partnership and stressful situations with the child. 1948 at a "Conference on Family Life", a two-dimensional scheme was presented: Developmental

tasks of children were one dimension, possible difficulties in the family associated with the child's different developmental stages the other.

Whereas the original concept of family developmental tasks centred on single stages during children's development and focused on the description of adequate activities of parent and children, newer approaches dealing with family development tend to emphasise time segments during development different from the single stages, they now focus on the transitions between two developmental stages. Here, during these passages where a well-established balance of living with a child of a certain developmental level has been lost or given up and where a new way of family life which is adapted to the child's next level of development has not yet been reached, crises are more likely and misunderstandings among family members may increase. It is the time of crisis management, and families have different strategies to master these periods, they vary according to their transition competence. Reuben Hill (1949) published the first version of a "family stress model" in which he illustrated the emergence of crises in the family and how to avoid them. The so-called ABCX model is still the prototype for a scheme to describe the various components of a family crisis.

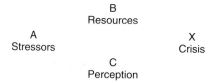

Fig. 2.1: ABCX Model for Family Stress after Reuben Hill (1948)

Under a family systems perspective, this model has been further elaborated, for example, by David Reiss in 1981 or by McCubbin and Patterson in 1983. The model shows four components: A is the stressor, the factors or the situation which initiates specific activities of the family members to cope with the stress. B represents the access to resources which can help to reduce stress, for example, easy or difficult access to expert advice, etc. C indicates the family's perception of the stressful situation. It is the interpretation of what emerges as a threatening event or what is seen as a kind of routine situation which can easily be resolved. A crying child, for instance, can be perceived by parents as a normal event and they know that there are enough resources available for them to master this situation. They take up the child, they know how to soothe it, and if all their attempts are unsuccessful, they see a doctor. It is no crisis at all. In another family, a crying child may symbolise all the restrictions the parents have had to suffer since the child arrived, it may represent the bleak outlook into the future, and the parents have no access to effective resources to find a way out of these confined conditions in family life.

In sum, relationship quality, sensitivity to development, and coping skills in transition represent major aspects that have been brought up more and more in recent years in developmental psychology in the light of results which emphasise the importance of relationship quality for infant and adolescent development. Moreover, these newer approaches mirror attempts to merge family and individual development, they also characterise what is believed to be essential for a child's proximal environment as they take account of the complexity of the family's relational network and add developmental dynamics to the static view of family interaction structures.

2.5 The parents' responsibility for producing a model for the maintenance of family relationships and the adaptation to children's developmental steps

The concept of family development emphasises not only environmental arrangements in the house to meet the needs of the growing children and the ageing parents, it also focuses on relational aspects that have been described by Rodgers (1973) as the maintenance of meaning and motivation in the family. Recent studies have shown that not only the quality of the parent-child relationship but also the quality of the relationship between both parents has an impact on the children's course of development. As an example, Emery (1982, 1988) found in a metaanalysis of different studies that children of pre-school and school age from families with conflict marital relationships show more problems in academic achievement and in establishing social relationships with peers than children from harmonious families. Moreover, Cummings et al. (1989) and Fainsilber-Katz & Gottman (1993) showed that when marital relationship is characterised not by aggression but by paternal withdrawal, children display low self-esteem and high anxiety. In another metaanalysis, Erel & Burman (1995) illuminated that there is a "spill-over effect" from the parent-parent to the parent-child relationship. This means that the quality of the parental relationship is replicated in the parent-child relationship. When parents cooperate and support each other when caring for the child, these children then develop higher coping abilities. (Belsky, Crnic, & Gable, 1995). Even during adolescence the quality of relationship seems to be important for the child's self development (Harold & Conger, 1997; Davies & Cummings, 1998).

Infants develop rapidly through various stages during the early years. Never again will the individual run through such a sequence of changes in such a short time as during the first 24 or 30 months. On all relevant developmental functions, from locomotoric to sensorimotoric and cognitive development, from affective and social to self development, the infant experiences a variety of fundamental changes, from a helpless, speechless, static and dependent human being to a full-fledged family member who is socially competent, who can walk and who understands language. During this phase of early development, parents have to adapt to the child's changing needs on the one hand, they have to socialise the child and to convey rules and norms to integrate the new member into the family's relational network on the other.

Furthermore, during the transition from partnership to parenthood, the parents themselves run through a difficult phase of mutual adaptation. The arrival of a child not only enlarges the number of persons in a family, it also changes the relational structure. Instead of a single dyad there are now three dyads, of which two are totally new and have to be established and maintained in the family. Moreover, the marital relationship has to be reorganised.

By establishing new relationships with the child, both parents experience new characteristics in the partner. Here perhaps unknown details of the other's personality may come to the fore. Cowan and Cowan (1987, 1992) have described this transition process as a dance, the "parental gavotte," where partners push and pull each other. Mothers sometimes become exhausted and experience the child as a stressful task. When they call on the father to participate in child care activities, they do not allow him to do it differently. If this pattern is repeated several times, it becomes frustrating for the partner and he withdraws from helping in childcare. In turn, this may create bad feelings in the mothers of being abandoned by their husbands, and so on.

When a second child is born in the family, changes in the relationship network become even more marked. Now the dyadic structure changes from a unit with three dyads to one with six dyads, from a unit with one triad to one with now four triads.

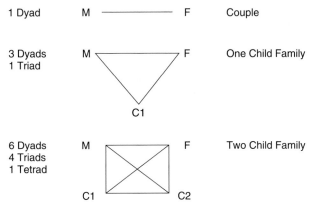

Fig. 2.2: Structural changes in families with one and two children

During the period after the arrival of a second child, families try to integrate the new child and at the same time to maintain or restructure the relationship with the first child. As the mother is – at least during the first months – preoccupied with the new child, the father becomes a crucial partner for the first child.

Generally, families have to go through quite a number of major transitions during the first two or three years in the life of a child, when crucial developmental shifts occur. For example, at 4/5 months, at 8/9 months, at 14/16 months and at 18/21 months fundamental developmental changes have to be accompanied and worked through by the parents. If these developmental steps are ignored or repressed, the developmental process of the child might be interrupted or a single function encapsulated, leading to problems during later developmental steps. Parental ignorance with regard to developmental changes and the lack of adaptation to new needs and skills of the child may have a major negative impact on the functioning of the entire family as a developing unit. For example, the onset of the understanding of language in the child is seen by most parents as a dramatic turning point in their strategy of socialising. As the frequency diagram from a longitudinal study with families with a child during the first 24 months shows, parents do change their socialising behaviour drastically according to perceived developmental progress (Kreppner, 1988, 1991). New abilities of the child become visible between 8 and 12 months, and the intentional exploration of the world of objects, the testing of affective reactions of the parents as well as the growing ability to understand language bring to the fore new parental demands for the child. Parents drastically begin to convey rules and norms in order to integrate their child into the framework of habits and rituals of the family.

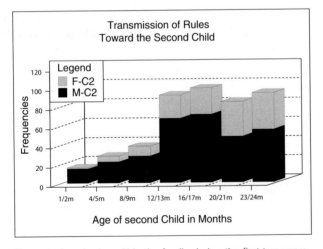

Fig. 2.3: Transmission of rules within the family during the first two years

These mutual adaptations are always potential crises and have to be mastered by all family members. Changes of behaviour in one member and new demands alter the actual relationship balance and therefore create stress. From a family developmental perspective, these phases are periods of disorganisation where new modes of living together have to be established. The mastering of these normative transition crises has been labelled as a specific skill, as a basic characteristic of family functioning, and as an important element for the quality of a child's developmental pathway (Cowan, 1991).

2.6 Differences in dealing with crises during family developmental transitions

The transition from partnership to parenthood always has a heavy impact on family well-being, as the study of Olson and McCubbin (1983) has shown. In this large cross-sectional study covering families of all stages during the life span, marital communication declined and consideration of divorced increased dramatically after the arrival of children in young families. Do we have indicators for factors that show how these transition crises can be mastered? Of course, developmental progress in the child can be handled by families in different ways. Parents may experience developmental changes in their child as enrichment or threat. They may ignore changes and new demands of their child and then find themselves in stressful situations where old routines of living together break up and no longer function as they did before. However, new and more appropriate regulations that could cope with the child's developmental progress have not yet been developed or negotiated among family members.

Rapid transitions do not only occur during the early years in family life. Later, when children reach adolescence, changes in the child are again very dramatic. Families vary considerably in their capacities to meet the new demands for autonomy as well as in their abilities to guide the child appropriately into adulthood. Adaptation of relationships and patterns of communication between parents and adolescents from a child-oriented to an adult-oriented format can be identified as a general family-developmental task during this transition period. Divergent patterns of communication quality within the families were revealed in a study comparing three groups of adolescents who had assessed their relationship quality with their parents constantly over a three and a half year period as "secure", "habitual" or "ambivalent" (for details see Kreppner & Ullrich, 1998). Families were classified according to adolescents' judgements and marked differences were found, for example, with regard to important non-verbal aspects of everyday communication such as the production of closeness during discussions in all family dyads. High closeness was characteristic for all dyadic communications in families where adolescents had judged their relationship with the parents as secure and satisfying, low closeness was consistently found in families with adolescents who had assessed the quality of their relationship with their parents as being ambivalent.

In another study (Kreppner 2001, 2002), communication patterns within the families were compared for two groups of adolescents where adolescents had changed their assessments about their well being in the family over time in quite different directions. In one group, adolescents judged their own well-being in the family as getting better and better, in the other worse and worse.

Here, again not only parent-child but particularly parent-parent communication patterns showed huge differences between the two groups. In the group of adolescents

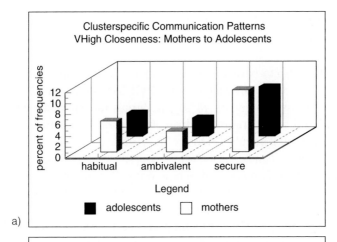

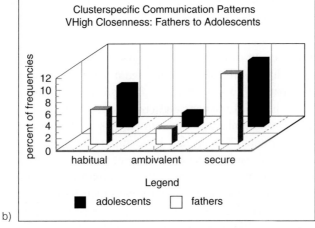

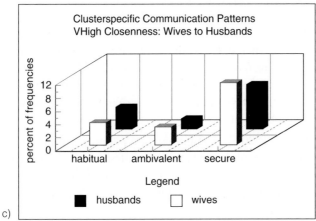

Fig. 2.4: Clusterspecific differences (habitual, ambivalent, and secure) in "very high" closeness across the three family dyads mother-adolescent (a), father-adolescent (b), and husband-wife (c)

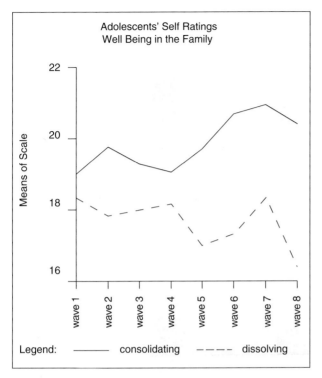

Fig. 2.5: Different assessments of well being in change groups

where the feeling of well-being in the family increased over time, parents showed more integrative behaviour than the parents in the other group, they also differed in the degree of closeness in their dyadic communications.

These results not only point to the fact that clear indicators exist which can characterise different relational and emotional conditions in families, where adolescents either feel well or do not, but also specifically suggest that the quality of the parent-parent communications can be taken as a strong indicator for a family's likelihood to deal successfully with transition periods in childhood and adolescence.

2.7 Considerations about how to communicate knowledge about family health

Communication of knowledge about factors that are relevant for family well-being and family health should focus on central issues in individual and family development such as basic developmental changes during childhood and adolescence, relationship quality in the family, and mastering of transition crises. In such a list of

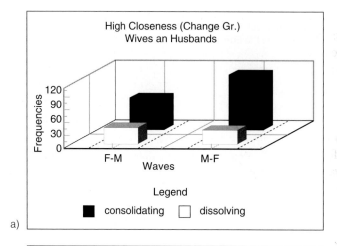

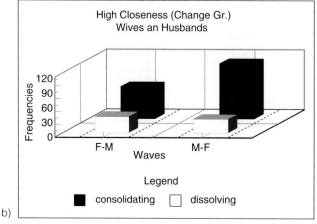

Fig. 2.6: Closeness (a) and integration (b) in parental communication (change groups)

basic knowledge about what is important to keep a family together, dynamics of family life and necessary steps of adaptation to developmental changes in the child should be elaborated in detail. The art of reorganising ill-functioning relationships could be another topic in that list. Furthermore, a guide for young parents should also include information about how to get access to a variety of resources which might help prevent the emergence of crises and convey security when parents are confronted with normative developmental shifts in the family.

Teaching and transmission of basic knowledge about how to run a functioning and satisfying relationship cannot be too early in childhood. Parents can convey communication competence to their children at a very early age, during language acquisition and before, and children can learn about normative developmental crises in family life and reflect their experiences as early as in kindergarten and school. By the same token, during early adulthood, whenever families are founded and partners become parents, basic knowledge about establishing, maintaining, and negotiating a relationship should be available. As Cowan and Cowan (1992) have nicely shown in their study about the management of problems during the transition to parenthood, intervention is possible and has a positive effect: Young families who had the opportunity to participate in guided meetings with other young parents, for example, showed lower divorce rates than young couples who had no such opportunity. Sometimes public institutions, counselling centres, and administrations seem to offer plenty of detailed information about the course of children's development, about possible sicknesses, ways to optimise children's physical environments, and so forth. In most cases, however, the agenda does not include the parents' own needs during this period, or techniques for the integration of the child in the family's specific framework. Family-specific aspects of how to maintain and reorganise a relationship during the life span are often totally neglected.

Three aspects of internal family functioning were elaborated in this contribution: Family as a developing unit, the art of relationship maintenance, and, the importance of the parent-parent relationship as a model of communication for the child. Being a competent parent also implies sensitivity for and good knowledge about developmental steps in the child. It may be true that the necessity to reorganise formats of family life during specific periods may create crises, but it is always possible to find a way out. Ignorance of developmental changes and stagnation in family relationships may lead to pathological developmental pathways, whereas active work to find a new common basis for living together during times of transition should be taken as a healthy sign.

2.8 References

[1] Aldous, J. (1978). Family careers. New York: Wiley.
[2] Belsky, J., Crnic, K., & Gable, S. (1995). The determinants of coparenting in families with toddler boys: Spousal differences and daily hassles. Child Development, 66, 629–642.
[3] Cowan, P. A. (1991). Individual and family life transitions: A proposal for a new definition. In P. A. Cowan & M. Hetherington, (eds.), Family transitions, (pp. 3–30). Hillsdale, NJ: Lawrence Erlbaum.
[4] Cowan, C. P. & Cowan, P. A. (1992). When partners become parents: The big life change for couples. New York: Basic Books.
[5] Cowan, C. P., & Cowan, P. A. (1987). Men's involvement in parenthood: Identifying the antecedents and understanding the barriers. In P. W. Berman & F. A. Pedersen (Eds.), Men's transition to parenthood (pp. 145–174). Hillsdale, NJ: Lawrence Erlbaum.
[6] Cummings, J. S., Pellegrini, D. S., Notarius, C. I., & Cummings, E. M. (1989). Children's responses to angry adult behaviour as a function of marital distress and history of interparental hostility. Child Development, 60, 1035–1043.
[7] Davies, P. T. & Cummings, E. M. (1998). Exploring children's security as a mediator of the link between marital relations and child adjustment. Child Development, 69, 124–139.

 [8] Duvall, E. (1977). Marriage and family development. New York: Lippincott.

 [9] Duvall, E. & Hill, R. (1945). When you marry. New York: Association Press.

[10] Emery, R. E. (1988). (Ed.). Marriage, divorce, and children's adjustment. Newbury Park, CA: Sage.

[11] Emery, R. E. (1982) Interparental conflict and the children of discord and divorce. Psychological Bulletin, 92, 310−330.

[12] Erel, O. & Burman, B. (1995). Interrelatedness of marital and parent-child relations: A meta-analytic review. Psychological Bulletin, 118, 108−13.

[13] Fainsilber-Katz, L. & Gottman, J. M. (1993). Patterns of marital conflict predict children's internalising and externalising behaviours. Developmental Psychology, 29, 940−950.

[14] Gottman, J. M., Fainsilber-Katz, L., & Hooven, C. (1996) Meta-emotion: How families communicate emotionally. Mahwah, NJ: Erlbaum.

[15] Harold, G. T. & Conger, R. D. (1997). Marital conflict and adolescent distress: The role of adolescent awareness. Child Development, 68, 333−350.

[16] Havighurst, R. J. (1948). Developmental tasks and education. New York: McKay.

[17] Hill, R. (1949). Families under stress. New York: Harper & Row.

[18] Kreppner, K. (2002). Retrospect and prospect in the psychological study of families as systems. In J. McHale & W. Grolnick (Eds.), Retrospect and prospect in the psychological study of families (pp. 225−257). Mahwah, NJ: Erlbaum.

[19] Kreppner, K. (2001). Variations in children's perceived relationship quality and changes in communication behaviors within the family during the child's transition to adolescence: A differential approach. In J. R. M. Gerris (Editor) Dynamics of Parenting (pp.33−52). Leuven: Garant.

[20] Kreppner, K. (1991). Observation and the longitudinal approach in infancy research. In M. Lamb & H. Keller (Eds.), Infant development: Perspectives from German-speaking countries (pp. 151−178). Hillsdale, NJ: Lawrence Erlbaum.

[21] Kreppner, K. (1988). Changes in dyadic relationships within a family after the arrival of a second child. In R. A. Hinde & J. Stevenson-Hinde (Eds.), Relationships within families: Mutual influences. (pp. 143−167). Oxford: Oxford University Press.

[22] Kreppner, K. & Ullrich, M. (1998). Talk to mom and dad, and listen to what is in between. In M. Hofer, P. Noack, & J. Youniss, (Eds.), Verbal interaction and development in families with adolescents (pp. 83−108). Greenwich, CT: Ablex.

[23] McCubbin, H. I. & Patterson, J. M. (1983). The family stress process: The double ABCX model of adjustment and adaptation. Marriage and Family Review, 6, 7−37.

[24] Olson, D. H. & McCubbin, H. I. (1983). Families. London: Sage Publication.

[25] Reiss, D. (1981). The family's construction of reality. Cambridge Mass.: Harvard. University Press.

[26] Rodgers, R. (1973). Family interaction and transaction. The developmental approach. Englewood Cliffs, NJ: Prentice Hall.

[27] Sorce, J. F., Emde, R. N., Campos, J., & Klinnert, M. D. (1985). Maternal emotional signaling: Its effect on the visual cliff behaviour of 1-year-olds. Developmental Psychology, 21, 195−200.

[28] Trevarthen, C. & Hubley, P. (1978). Secondary intersubjectivity: Confidence, confinding and acts of meaning in the first year. In A. Lock (Ed.), Action, gesture and symbol (pp. 183−229). London: Academic Press.

[29] Tronick, E. Z. (1989). Emotions and emotional communication in infants. American Psychologist, 44, 112−119.

[30] Tronick, E. Z. & Cohn, J. (1989). Infant-mother face-to-face interaction: Age and gender differences in coordination and the occurrence of miscoordination. Child Development, 60, 85−91.

[31] Vives, J. L. (1531;1913). On education. Translation of De tradendis disciplinis, from De disciplinis libri XX (1531) by F. Watson. Cambridge: Cambridge University Press.

2.9 Discussion

Prof. Brodehl (Chair):
... do you want to make a comment first? Not the case at the moment. So please, who wants to ask questions or discuss. Dr Manz please.

Dr. Manz:
There is a clear change in the kind of professional perception and professional advice. If we look what (the) paediatrician told parents during this century, there (is a dramatic change). And this is: the population does not always know the newest (ideas), and even within the profession there is a clear generational gap and so on. So I think you should comment on this.

Dr. Kreppner:
Could you elaborate a bit on the generational gap, what do you mean?

Prof. Manz:
Oh, there is a book of Czerny in 1908: "Der Arzt als Erzieher des Kindes". And if you look at this, the parents address the doctor. And Czerny was realizing it in 1905 And so we should think about our advice ourselves.

Dr. Kreppner:
I think that we had this kind of advice from James Watson[*] for example in the twenties, that parents should not be too warm to their children because this is bad for the children and all this stuff, going back to conditioning... I think we had a big break-through in the seventies, in this kind of area where ethologists began to observe small children, infants in interaction with their mothers, and what is going on in this relationship, and how important this is. And I think from that time on it has made progress, even in hospitals, and so we had rooming-in, that the children stay with the mothers, and we had of course more information in the direction that I alluded to. But still I think it is not enough. What we found in the last twenty years is the importance of the marital relationship in the family for the developmentof the children. This had not been touched upon. Normally, of course we know this somehow, but there are systematic studies now about the association between the quality of relationship of the parents and the healthy development of the children.

Prof. Dittmann:
Do you know about studies if the paediatricians are in front or behind regarding this quality of relationship?

---

[*] Watson, J. B. (1928). *Psychological care of infant and child.* New York: Norton.

Dr. Kreppner:
What I know is that there are huge differences. There are very progressive doctors who know about this. But this is not a kind of institutionalised knowledge, I think, so what I see is huge, huge differences about how to approach what it is important for the child's development. And so we have made progress during the seventies, I would say, but it is not enough.

Prof. Dittmann:
Are there systematic studies which show how doctors are approaching these programmes, and − because young parents are young and they are in front in understanding and so on, and the doctors are really old sometimes and so −

Prof. Brodehl:
[laughingly:] They keep to their own, so old!

Prof. Dittmann:
Old in experience. And therefore my question is: is there any study looking at how the professional situation is, are they ahead or behind?

Dr. Kreppner:
Perhaps someone here in the audience knows, I have no knowledge about this kind of special question and systematic studies about it. But it is an interesting question. [laughing:] You are doing this work, are you?

Prof. Brodehl (Chair):
Does somebody know? Herr Wolke, please.

Prof. Wolke:
Well I think, when I later talk about crying, feeding, and sleeping problems, there is an example: one of the big problems is that the needs of parents and the education like in medical school are completely apart. You see, parents are much less interested in how you take blood, how you do minor surgery, how you do particular things, but that is what you learn in hospital, what you do a lot of the time. Now they then suddenly become practitioners, where they work outside, where they are not using these procedures, because they refer them to the hospital because the junior doctors will be doing that. And I think that is the problem, it is more than just a generation problem: it is a problem that the training for a hospital doctor, for someone who is actually able to manage accidents, to manage on the ward, who takes blood, who does the screening. And actually, in the community, most of the time is actually spent talking about worries the parents have. I mean you still have to give advice on immunisation etc., but a lot of the problems which are related to the family, to particular behaviour problems that children have, are actually not delivered to medical school, and I think there has to be the major change: if you want to be a practitioner, a quite different approach.

Prof. Brodehl (Chair):
Thank you. Yes, Frau Bergmann?

Dr. Bergmann:
I think in the annual meeting of our professions, we always find that lectures dealing with this are full, totally crowded because doctors are so interested to learn about it. So the teacher, the doctor has to be taught first, before he can teach parents. There is really a lack of knowledge. When you talk, probably the auditorium is full!

Prof. Brodehl:
[laughing:] We will wait and see. Any further comment on this problem? No.

3 Frequent problems in infancy and toddler years: Excessive crying, sleeping and feeding difficulties

Dieter Wolke

3.1 Introduction

Excessive crying, often called "colic crying", sleep problems and feeding problems represent a considerable workload for primary health professionals and paediatricians. However, there are only few systematic reviews on origins, co-occurrence and treatment of these infancy problems. This chapter provides an overview of the normal development of fussing and crying, sleep regulation and feeding, identification and diagnosis of excessive crying, problems of initiating or maintaining sleep, as well as feeding and eating problems. Furthermore, it explores whether these difficulties are separate entities or often occur together (co-morbidity). Etiological factors, and factors that maintain cry, sleep and feeding problems will be identified and it will be investigated whether there are any long-term consequences of regulatory problems. Finally, an approach to the treatment of crying and sleeping problems as well as feeding problems will be outlined.

3.2 Crying, Sleeping and Feeding Problems: Definition and Prevalence

3.2.1 Excessive Crying

Fussing and crying duration shows a typical pattern over the first year of life in the normal new-born (Barr, 1990; Wolke, 1997a, St. James-Roberts & Halil, 1991) and healthy preterm infant (Barr et al., 1996)

- Cry duration increases from about 1.75 hours per day to about 2.5 hours until the 6th week of life
- Cry duration reduces to about 1 hour by the 4th month of life and then stabilises at this level until the end of the 1st year of life.
- About 40% of all infants in the first 3 months of life cry most between 4 pm and 11 pm (e. g. Walker & Menahem, 1994; St James Roberts & Halil, 1991).
- Excessive crying, often also labelled "colic crying", is defined by increased duration of crying. The most widely accepted definition is the rules of three: Crying

and fussing for more than 3 hours a day, for more than 3 days a week for the last 3 weeks (Wessel et al., 1954).

Other clinical symptoms such as frequently passing wind, clenching fists, drawn up legs, holding body straight etc. are often described in paediatric books and by parents, but are only occasionally co-occurring symptoms (Field, 1994). About 10–20 % of parents report excessive crying in the first months of life (St James Roberts & Halil, 1991; Lehtonen & Korvenranta, 1995). The onset of crying problems is thus usually within the first 2 months of life (Table 3.1).

3.2.2 Sleeping problems

Major changes in the physiological organisation of sleep, the circadian (day/night) and ultradian (within the day) rhythm and in the duration of sleep and waking are found within the 1st year of life (Wolke, 1994; Wolke, 1997). Circadian sleep/wake organisation is already noticeable in the 1st weeks of life with an increasing placing of the longest period of sleep during the night (Walker & Menaham, 1994, Bamford et al., 1990). The differentiation into active sleep (REM), light sleep (NREM, states 1, 2) and deep sleep (NREM states, 3, 4) starts in the first months of life and differentiation of the sleep stages is completed at the end of the 1st year. While newborns start their sleep with REM sleep, falling asleep from the 4th to the 6th months is initiated in non-REM sleep. A summary of the physiological sleep changes are to be found in table 3.2 (for more detail see Wolke (1994)).

- At the age of 6–8 months the sleep of an infant is structurally very similar to the sleep of the adult. However, infants and toddlers have multiple sleep phases during the day (naps).
- The sleep duration reduces from about 14–16 hours in the new-born to about 12–13 hours in the 2-year-old.

Toddlers and pre-schoolers are mainly reported of having problems in initiating and maintaining sleep (falling asleep and night-waking problems). Strictly speaking, these problems often represent distress caused to the parents by long evening rituals and waking at night. All infants wake 3 to 7 times per night, as has been demonstrated by infra red video somnography. However, the parents are only aware of this when the child cries or comes into their bed and the parents are woken and need to console the child (Minde et al., 1993; Gaylor et al., 1998). Children are not born with the ability to sleep through the night. Frequent awakening is adaptive to allow for frequent nutritional intake and to promote growth in the first 6 months of life (Wolke et al., 1998a; Skuse et al., 1994a).

- Night waking is defined as follows: the child wakes more than 5 nights per week at least once a night (between midnight and 5.00 a.m.) and is more than 6 months of age.

Table 3.1: Comparison of Excessive Crying-, Sleeping- and Feeding Problems: Symptoms

	Excessive Crying	Sleeping Problem	Feeding Problem
Onset	early/1.−2. month	1st year/any time	newborn/4−6 months
Prevalence			
Total	9−26%	15−25%	15−25%
Severe	5−10%	10%	5−10%
Co-morbidity	high	low/moderate	low/moderate (?)

Table 3.2: Sleep architecture and temporal pattern of sleep from infancy to adulthood:

	Infant	Adult
1) Sleep onset states	REM sleep onset	NREM sleep onset
2) Sleep state proportions		
a) REM/NREM (%)	40−45/55−60	20−25/75−80
b) Percentage of stage 4 sleep of total sleep	stage 3/4 discrimination − not established (children: 20−25%)	15−20%
3) Periodicity of sleep states	50−65 min. REM/NREM cycle	90−100 min. REM/NREM cycle
4) Day sleep	infants: polyphasic with several naps during day; 3−4 years of age loss of daytime nap	no daytime sleep
5) Temporal organization of sleep during night sleep	Infants: REM-NREM cycles equally distributed through night; predominance of NREM sleep in 1st third of night from 6 mths (i.e. children)	NREM stages 3−4 predominant 1st third of night; REM state predominant in last third of night
6) Development of EEG-pattern	Newborn: 1 NREM sleep stage Emergence of sleep NREM spindles: 4−8 weeks K-complex: 6−24 mths Delta-activity: 4−6 mths	4 NREM stages
7) Awakenings during the night	Infants: frequent (5−7 times) children: low (0−3 times) and short	low (0−2 times)

EEG: electroencephalogram; NREM: non-rapid eye movement; REM: rapid eye movement

- Severe night waking problems are defined when the child wakes up more than once per night;
- Falling asleep problems are defined as a) problems of settling routine, i. e. the child takes longer than an hour from the time of being asked to go to bed until the time it settles in bed or b) the child is in bed and takes longer than half an hour to fall asleep or c) need the parents to be present until asleep.

The prevalence of night waking problems is around $20-25\%$ in the first 2 years of life and around $7-13\%$ in the pre-school years (Stores, 1996; Wolke 1994; Wolke et al. 1994a; 1995b; 1998) (see table 3.1). Problems around sleeping routines or bed time routines are most prevalent in children of about $4-5$ years of age (Wolke 1994) (prevalence: $15-50\%$). Similarly, problems with falling asleep also show an increase from infancy to kindergarten age (around $9-12\%$) and stabilise during the school years and often show a renewed increase in adolescence Wolke, 1994; Wolke et al., 1994b).

3.2.3 Feeding and eating problems

Fluids are the major nutritional intake of all healthy new-borns and are provided either via breast or bottle. Between the age of $3-6$ months most infants are intro-duced to solid nutrition and between $9-15$ months infants show a tendency to feed themselves, first with their hands and then using utensils such as a spoon (Wolke Skuse, 1992, Wolke 1994). The prerequisites for successful feeding are (Skuse & Wolke 1992; Drewett et al., 1998).

- Anatomical maturation of the nervous system and muscular structures
- The development of appropriate oral motor abilities (from lip closure to chewing)
- Appropriate positioning and body posture during feeding
- Appropriate parent-child interaction.

A number of surveys have estimated that about 0.4% to 3% of all paediatric hospital admissions are related to severe feeding problems (Wolke, 1994). Roughly between 1.4% to 3% of severe feeding problems are diagnosed by those working in primary care and about $20-25\%$ of parents report about problems feeding infants in first 2 years (Lindberg et al., 1991) (Table 3.1). The most frequent problems in the first 6 months of life are:

- Daily vomiting $(3-6\%)$
- Food refusal (3%)
- Refusal of solid foods $(4-5\%)$
- Little appetite $(1-2\%)$
- Swallowing problems (1%)

Other problems that have been identified are difficulties with weaning (about 5%) (Drewett et al., 1998). Less severe problems such as transient difficulties with breastfeeding are not included in these prevalence estimates (Wolke & Skuse 1992). The most frequent feeding problems after the first 6 months of life are (Table 3.1):

- Refusal of most foods (approximately 3%)
- Refusal of solid food (approximately 4%)
- Lack of appetite (approximately 3%)

In about half of the cases food refusers show growth retardation, i.e. these children show growth patterns substantially below those of normal eaters (Lindberg, 1994). A further diagnosis, *failure to thrive,* is frequent, but is often not associated with obvious eating disorders (Drewett et al., 1999; Dowdney et al., 1987; Heptinstall et al., 1987; Wilensky et al., 1996; Skuse et al., 1992, Ramsey, 1995). There are several definitions of failure to thrive, either related to growth rate or to attained weight. A frequent definition in community studies is

- A child shows a relative weight loss compared to peers below 1.88 standard deviations (below the 3rd weight percentile) in the first 2 years of life although born at normal birth weight (Skuse et al., 1994b).

The prevalence of failure to thrive is about $3-4\%$ in infancy and toddler populations (Wolke et al., 1990; Skuse et al., 1994a, b; Wilensky et al., 1996; Drewett et al., 1999).

Feeding problems can occur at any time during infancy and the pre-school years starting with the newborn, at the time of introduction of solid food $(4-6$ months) and during later introduction of foods that make high demands on oral motor skills, for example, the introduction of meat or dried foods which require complex chewing. Weight loss can occur at any time, but it has been suggested to be most detrimental to brain development and long-term cognitive development if it occurs in the first 6 months of life (Skuse et al., 1994a). However, recent research on infants in Ethiopia growing up in highly deprived nutritional conditions indicates that malnutrition at any time during the first 2 years of life has detrimental effects on brain development and cognitive abilities.

3.2.4 Co-morbidity of crying, sleeping and feeding problems

Greenspan and Lourie (1981) and de Gangi et al. (1991) suggested that infants and toddlers $(0-3$ years) suffer a regulatory disturbance if at least 2 of 4 symptoms are present: hyper-excitability, difficulty to calm themselves (excessive crying or repeated tantrums), sleep or feeding problems. Regulatory disturbance has been suggested as a primary disturbance in the diagnostic classification of mental health and developmental disorders of infancy and early childhood (DC: $0-3$) (Zero to Three 1994; Thomas and Clark, 1998). Only in recent years have there been empirical investigations of the co-occurrence and the relationships between different infancy behaviour problems (von Hofacker & Papousek 1998; Wolke et al. 1994b; 1995a; 1998; McDonough et al., 1998). It has been suggested that the core symptoms of regulatory disturbance are crying, sleeping and feeding problems.

Two studies on clinical populations of children aged 1−6 months who were referred for excessive crying (on average 4.5 for 6 hours crying per day) reported that these children also have significant sleep disturbances or feeding problems in a majority of cases (von Hofacker & Papousek, 1996; Wolke et al., 1994b). Wolke et al. (1994b) reported that approximately 80% of parents of excessive criers who had sought help from professionals also reported feeding problems and 70% sleeping problems in their infants. Von Hofacker and Papousek (1998) also found that 77% of excessive criers had sleeping problems and 34% had feeding problems. Altogether, about 58% had a secondary disturbance and 23% had excessive crying, sleeping and feeding problems. Less co-association between crying and sleeping problems was found in this study between 7 and 12 months and 13 to 24 months. However, the von Hofacker and Papousek (1998) clinical population still had problems in more than one domain in 47−64% of cases.

A prospective population study showed that about 40−50% of all children had more than one type of problem (Wolke et al., 1995b). However, only 1.9% of children had problems in all three areas (see table 3.1). Lindberg et al. (1991) further found some co-association of vomiting with crying problems. The limited evidence so far indicates a co-association of problems and that co-morbidity is more frequent in clinical populations. It appears that parents with multiple problems are more likely to seek professional help.

There is a lack of studies that have concerned themselves with the mechanisms and diagnostic importance of co-morbidity crying, sleeping and feeding difficulties (Wolke, 1995a). Crying and night-waking appear to be important mechanisms of regulation of nutritional intake in young infants. Children who start sleeping through the night within the first weeks of life and are not awoken by their parents for feeds appear to have an increased risk for failure to thrive (Skuse et al., 1994a). Children who cry more are more likely to be fed more frequently and grow better (Carey, 1986). There appears to be an inverted U-type relationship between cry and waking behaviour whereby moderate crying and waking in the first months of life is adaptive to secure physical closeness, adequate feeding and normal growth. Infants who cry little are at increased risk of being ignored, receiving less social stimulation and less nutrition, while too much crying and too frequent night-waking can lead to exhaustion and distress in the parents and to adverse consequences such as child abuse if paired with parents who have little resources (shaken baby syndrome) (Frodi, 1985; Zeskind & Shingler, 1991).

3.3   Etiological factors

3.3.1 Child-related factors

Children who either cry excessively, have sleep problems or are food refusers are often reported by their parents to have a difficult temperament (Wolke & St James

Robert, 1987; Wolke et al., 1990; 1994b; Lindberg, 1994; Lindberg et al. 1996; Scher et al. 1992; Carey, 1990; Atkinson et al., 1995) (table 3.3). Children who are later identified as excessive criers appear to be more active already in utero (St James Roberts, 1999) or to show increased irritability in the first days of life (van den Boom, 1988). Differences in physiological reactivity have been documented in children with regulatory disturbances, for example in vagal tone, (De Gangi et al., 1991; Lewis, 1992). Recent investigations that employed direct observation of temperament characteristics and objective recordings of sleeping (video-somnography; for example Halpern, et al., 1994; Keener et al., 1988) have indicated moderate associations between sleep indices and temperament. Difficult temperament (high reactivity, low self regulation, negative emotionality) appears to indicate or reflect poorer self-regulation of the infant. A range of recent studies have indicated that the major difficulty of children with crying and sleeping problems is not necessarily increased reactivity (i. e. they do not cry more frequently), but that they lack self-regulation (St James Roberts 1991). Difficult temperament is an important factor shaping the behaviour of parents and of the social environment (Owen-Stively et al., 1997).

Physical problems and biological risk factors (perinatal and neonatal complications) are rarely found to be predisposing factors for crying or sleeping problems or failure to thrive (Skuse et al., 1992; Lindberg, 1994; Haag & Dahl, 1987; Dahl & Sundelin 1986; Millar & Dahl, 1991; Messer & Richards, 1993). Crying and feeding problems, in particular oral motor dysfunctions are more frequently found in children with neurological problems, for example, very preterm born children (Wolke et al., 1994c; Skuse & Wolke, 1992; Riley et al., 1995, 1999). Although reported by some studies (Blurton-Jones et al., 1978), even severe prenatal and perinatal factors and prolonged hospitalisation or re-hospitalisation have little or no effect on the development of sleeping (McMillan et al., 1991) or the prevalence of sleeping problems (Ungerer et al., 1983; Tirosh et al., 1993; Wolke et al., 1995b, 1998). However, sleeping problems are found more frequently in children with severe developmental delay or severe learning disorders (Stores, 1996) (table 3.3). Cow milk protein intolerance as a pre-disposing factor for sleep, crying and feeding problems has been discussed both in the paediatric and popular literature (Lothar et al., 1982; Kahn et al., 1989). There is some evidence from randomized control trials that sub-groups may benefit from change of diets by breastfeeding mothers or changes in formulas in those who are bottle fed. Empirical studies, however, indicate that only 5−10% of crying or sleeping problems may be caused by transient cow milk protein intolerance, food allergy or other organic problems (American Academy of Paediatrics, 1989; Kahn et al., 1989; Wolke & Meyer, 1995; Lethonen, Gormally & Barr, in press).

3.3.2 Family and social factors

There are indications that sleeping problems (Messer & Richards, 1993; Messer & Parker, 1998) and excessive crying (Wolke et al., 1994b) are more frequent in families

Table 3.3: Comparison of Excessive Crying-, Sleeping- and Feeding Problems: Child Factors

	Excessive Crying	Sleeping Problem	Feeding Problem
Difficult temperament	moderate/strong	moderate	moderate
Organic problems	very rare	very rare	rare
Peri-, neonatal factors	no/rare	no	rare

where other siblings suffer behaviour problems. Feeding problems often run in families, for example, parents and siblings of feeding problems infants have more often had eating problems themselves (Lindberg, 1994; Dahl et al., 1986). It is unclear whether this may be explained by genetic or environmental transmission or both (Table 3.4).

When considering family and social factors as contributors of crying, sleeping or feeding disorder, it is important to distinguish between factors that predict the behaviour versus factors that relate to help seeking behaviour of parents. St James Roberts distinguished between actual behaviour and the impact it has on parents. Community studies have shown, somewhat surprisingly, that socio-demographic factors such as socio-economic status, education, age of the parents, number of siblings or birth order show no or only weak associations with all three disorders (St James Roberts, 1992; Lozoff and Zuckermann, 1988; Lindberg, 1994; Wolke, 1995a; Wolke & Messer, in press; Messer & Parker, 1998). In contrast, older mothers, first time mothers and those living in more affluent areas are more likely to seek help, for example, for colic problems (Table 3.4).

Table 3.4: Comparison of Excessive Crying-, Sleeping- and Feeding Problems: Family Factors

	Excessive Crying	Sleeping Problem	Feeding Problem
Family history	?	?	moderate
Sociodemographic	no/low	no/low	no/low
Social support	minor	minor	no/minor
Psychopathology of mother	yes	yes	yes

Social support does not appear to have a direct influence on crying, sleep or feeding problems (e. g. Lindberg, 1994; Messer & Richards, 1993) or influence maternal responsiveness (Owens & Shaw, 1998). Social support mainly influences how distressed the parents feel by the child's behaviour. Maternal depression and anxiety have repeatedly been shown to show a moderately strong relationship to sleep, crying and feeding problems (Zuckerman et al., 1987, 1990; Stoleru, 1997; Skuse and Wolke,1992; Wolke, 1990; Wolke et al., 1994c; Sarimski,1993).

It is unclear whether depressive symptoms and anxiety are a consequence of the behavioural symptoms of the child or a precursor. The evidence so far indicates that both may be the case. Millar et al. (1993) in their short-term prospective study showed that mothers of infants who became excessive criers within the first weeks of life did not differ in their depression scores during pregnancy. However, excessive crying during the first 6 weeks of life led to an increase in depression scores in the mothers. This indicates that the behaviour of infants may contribute to the development of psychopathology in the mother (Murray et al., 1996). On the other hand there is evidence that mothers who have been depressed previously (onset in adolescence) are much more likely to become depressed during pregnancy and in the postnatal period (Kurstjens & Wolke, in press). A range of studies have found that depressed mothers interact differently (i.e. they are more irritable, less attentive and less sensitive) with their infants (Murray).

3.4 Short and long-term consequences

The persistence of sleeping problems is moderate, i.e. a sleeping problem child is twice as likely to remain one as a non-sleeping problem child is to become one (Wolke et al., 1994a; 1995b; 1998; Jenkins et al., 1984). Children who cry more during the first 3 months of life show a tendency to also cry more later in the first year of life. However, the total duration of crying will decline in these early excessive criers. Children who have been diagnosed with food refusal or high food selectivity show a strong persistence of symptoms into middle childhood. Most of the children who were food refusers in the 1st year of life still show a much increased incidence of feeding problems in childhood (Dahl et al., 1994, Rydahl et al., 1995; Table 3.5).

Persistent somatic health problems related to sleeping and crying problems in early childhood or infancy have not been reported. In contrast, severe feeding problems in infancy are often associated with long-term growth and somatic problems such as anaemia and high susceptibility to infections. Approximately 50% of children with food refusal in infancy show failure to thrive (Dahl & Kristiansen, 1987; Lindberg, 1994). Poor growth as a symptom of undernutrition may lead to an infection/undernutrition cycle where the child often suffers infections that reduces nutritional intake even further which then leads to further infections and so on (Wolke, 1994). Recent community studies have indicated that stunted growth and low weight gain are the most frequent long-term complications of failure to thrive in infancy and the toddler years (Drewett et al., 1999).

No adverse effects on cognitive development have been reported for sleeping problems (Pollock, 1992) or excessive crying (Lethonen et al., in press; Wolke et al., 1997). In contrast, children who have been diagnosed with failure to thrive in infancy (with or without feeding problems), in particular, if failure to thrive is already present in the first 6 months of life, are at an increased risk for early cognitive developmental deficits and growth retardation (Wolke, 1994; Skuse et al., 1994b; Boddy, 1997; Dowdney et al., 1999). Since the original publication by Skuse et al. (1994b) of adverse effects of early growth retardation on cognitive development in the toddler years and early childhood, several studies have replicated the finding (Wilensky et al., 1996). However, the cognitive deficits may be confined to early childhood. A recent study by Drewett et al. (1999) indicated that children who fail to thrive appear to catch-up in cognitive abilities by middle to late childhood if their failure to thrive is not persistent.

There is some evidence that infants with crying, sleep or feeding problems are more likely to be hyperactive (Forsyth & Canny, 1991; Dahl & Sunderlin, 1992; Pollock, 1992; Stores, 1996). The association of early feeding problems with hyperactivity appears to be the strongest and best documented. Most of the follow-up on crying and sleeping problems have used parents' reports to assess behavioural consequences. There is controversy whether these reflect parental perceptions or observable child behaviour. Lethonen et al. showed that colic crying is relatively persistent over the first few months of life but that the prognosis for later behaviour, mother-child interaction or attachment problems is generally favourable, i. e. there are only small differences between colic and non-colic babies. Similarly, Barr's (1998) review of findings from 4 new follow-up studies of infants with prior colic found that most colicky infants show a significant reduction in the amount of crying over time, and their parents usually have intact relationships and are responsive to their infants. No more significant maternal distress and generally normal attachment relationships were reported. However, for a sub-group of infants, especially those from families with substantial additional risk factors, early excessive crying may evolve into a more generalised persistent mother-infant distress syndrome. In general, it appears that early crying problems affect the perception of mothers regarding behaviour problems, difficult temperament and family stress (Raihä et al., 1996). Wolke et al. (1995a) reported that the distress experienced by mothers predicted later development of sleeping problems in early childhood. A recent large longitudinal study of cry babies and their controls (N = 1348; birth to 9 years; Wolke & Meyer 1998) confirms the findings from smaller studies (Lethonen et al., in press; Barr, 1998). Crying problems within the first 5 months had no long-term effects on mother-child interaction at 6 and 8 years of age and only minor effects on observed child behaviour in achievement situations. However, mothers themselves reported more behaviour problems when they had an ex cry baby which may be explained by perception effects.

Early sleeping problems (before the 3rd year of life) generally show no relationship to later behavioural problems. However, with increasing age, sleeping problems are more often found in children with hyperactivity and anxiety problems and may also be related to problematic adaptation to school (Wolke, 1994; Stevenson, 1993; Caplan et al., 1987; Stores, 1996). Falling asleep and night waking problems are relatively unspecific symptoms in school age-children. They can indicate no behavioural problems, general behaviour problems, dysfunctional family relationships, or child abuse (Stores, 1996; Glod et al., 1997; see table 3.5).

Table 3.5: Comparison of Excessive Crying-, Sleeping- and Feeding Problems: Consequences

	Excessive Crying	Sleeping Problem	Feeding Problem
Persistence	low	moderate	high
Health problems (Infections, growth)	rare	no	moderate/strong
Cognitive development	no	no	yes, if FTT
Behaviour problems (Hyperactivity)	low	low	moderate
Mother-Child relationship (attachment, child abuse)	low/moderate	low/moderate	moderate
Social Interaction (across situations)	low	low	moderate

Feeding problems show a strong relationship to later insecure infant-mother attachment (Lindberg, 1994). There are conflicting results regarding the relationship of crying problems to later attachment relationships with their mothers. Neither Stifter and Bono (1998) nor Walker and Menahem (1994) found any negative effects on mother-child interactions or attachment relationship for ex-colicky infants. In contrast, van den Boom (1988) reported a significant relationship between early infant irritability and later insecure attachment. However, this relationship was only found if irritable infants had mothers with low caring competence who showed early patterns of mal-adaptive interaction with their infants. Thus, excessive crying problems may only show adverse effects on the mother-infant relationship if there are a range of other problems in the family including maternal depression (Papousek & von Hofacker, 1998).

Sagi et al. (1998) showed that frequent night waking showed significant relationships with insecure (ambivalent) attachment and lower maternal sensitivity in interaction with her child at 12 months of age. Benoit et al. (1992) further reported that mothers who have unresolved attachment relationships to their own parents, more frequently have children with sleeping problems. Maternal attachment representation correlates approximately 0.50 with child-mother attachment (van Ijzendoorn & Schingel, in press) The effects of infant problems on the infant-mother relationship are transgenerational via maternal behaviour (sensitivity in interaction) and due to particular challenges given by a difficult infant (Anders, 1994). Mothers who themselves experienced poor attachment representations may find it more difficult to let go of their infant at night time (settling to bed).

Cry and feeding problems have been further described as the last straw for child abuse (Frodi, 1985; Zeskind & Shingler, 1991). Parents who have abused their children often report that they could not cope with a continuous crying of their infant. They shook their baby, hit it or threw it into the bed, because they "just wanted their baby to shut up" (AAP, 1993).

Some generalisation of negative interaction styles in dealing with the problems of sleeping, feeding and crying to play behaviour have been suggested. These generalisations to play behaviour are small for sleeping problems (Minde et al., 1994), mild to moderate for crying problems (e. g. mothers who are often exhausted spend less time playing; Wolke & St James Roberts, 1987) and moderately high for feeding problems (Lindberg et al., 1996). However, children with sleeping problems are more often irritable and less attentive during the day (Minde et al., 1994).

To summarise, severe feeding problems such as food refusal during the 1st year of life have a number of adverse consequences, in particular, if there is also poor weight gain. These consequences include a high persistence of symptoms and adverse effects on cognitive, behavioural and social development (Wolke, 1994; Dowdney et al., 1987; 1999). Early excessive crying does not appear to have any adverse health consequences. Only in a minority of families that are already under stress are negative effects on mother-child interaction found. However, mothers of crying babies are more likely to perceive behaviour problems during the pre-school years which may reflect either biased perception or that the children do indeed behave differently towards their mothers than other people in their social network. Sleeping problems during the toddler years are not usually precursors of behaviour problems in childhood. However, all three regulatory problems appear to be related to insecure attachment of the child to the mother. Again, this may be more likely if the mother shows other psycho-social stress or psychological problems. Where such multiple infant and family problems are detected early in infancy, appropriate actions may help to prevent early physical abuse (AAP, 1993).

Although some have argued that early regulatory problems, i. e. the occurrence of a number of regulatory difficulties, may be related to long-term behavioural adaptation (van Hofacker & Papousek, 1998; De Gangi et al., 1991), few empirical studies have been conducted. Weissbluth (1987) proposed that many post-colic-children will develop sleeping problems. Wolke et al. (1995a) investigated whether a single problem (crying, sleeping or feeding) at 5 months provides a poorer prognosis than if the children had multiple problems. Children who had multiple problems at 5 months did not show sleeping problems more often at 20 and 56 months of age than children who only had sleeping problems at 5 months. Only those crying or feeding problem children who also showed frequent night waking at 5 months still had night waking problems more often at 20 or 56 months of age. This shows that excessive crying per se does not lead to more frequent sleeping problems or that multiple problems are indicative of a worse prognosis.

However, parents of children with multiple problems are often more distressed and are more likely to seek help from professionals (St James Roberts, 1992). Infants who show regulatory problems and have parents who have psychological problems are more likely to have long-term developmental problems (Papousek, 1999, Murray & Cooper, 1997; Esser, Laucht & Schmidt, 1994).

3.5 Summary

Excessive crying, sleeping and feeding problems occur together in about 1 case in 3. Severe regulatory problems (all 3 symptoms) are found in about 2% of infants in the population.

Sleeping problems can be considered as mainly influenced by early environmental entrainment (Wolke et al. 1998; Sarimski, 1993; MacMillan et al., 1991). In contrast, feeding problems usually present a particular challenge and are often related to minor organic problems or child factors ranging from lack of hunger and appetite to oral motor problems or hypersensitivity in the oral motor area (Mattison at al, 1998; Skuse & Wolke, 1992; Illingworth & Lister, 1964; Reilly et al., 1999). Crying problems occupy a middle position between sleeping and feeding problems in that they are both influenced by child characteristics such as difficult temperament and style of care. Multiple symptoms (regulatory problems) are more distressing for parents than the presence of just one problem. However, there is a lack of empirical data indicating that the prognosis for these children is worse. The clinical concept of regulatory disturbance is conceptionally, and heuristically helpful, however, different factors are related to each individual problem and the consequences differ. This makes it doubtful that they should be at this stage considered within one diagnostic category of regulatory problems (Barr, in press). Clinical samples indicate that mothers of regulatory disturbed infants and toddlers frequently suffer psychiatric problems (Papousek, 1999) and the infants often have minor neurological problems (Papousek & van Hofacker, 1998). The continuity of infancy problems are thus likely to be related to early minor neurological problems and persistent mother problems in interactions with her infant. These factors may lead to a vicious circle in some mother-infant dyads.

3.6 A model of factors that lead to and maintain infancy problems

A number of models have been proposed to explain the development or maintenance of regulatory problems. These include psycho-dynamic approach (e. g. Daws, 1989), strict behavioural approaches (e. g. Rickett and Johnson, 1988), behavioural-cognitive approaches (Wolke, 1996; France, 1996; Sarimski , 1993) or complex system models (Papousek & Papousek, 1996). Of these different models, behavioural management has received the most thorough empirical evaluation (see below). A behavioural management approach will be presented in the following (Wolke, 1996, Wolke et al. 1993).

Crying, sleeping and eating are primary biological needs. Crying is the first form of verbal communication, which is adaptive in an evolutionary sense by promoting survival and future reproductive success of the child. Lummaa, Wuorisalo, Barr and Lethonen (1998) and Wolke (1998) describe that crying increases closeness to the parents (e. g. carrying) and is likely to reduce the incidence of infanticide as intense crying indicates vigour of the infant. Furthermore, increased crying leads to more parental care as well as increased feeding in competition with siblings. Sleeping is necessary for the regeneration of the body and CNS and consolidates information processing of cognitive stimuli. Eating is a pre-requisite for central nervous system development and necessary for the immense physical growth required in the first year of life. During the 1st year of life growth (tripling of weight in first year alone) is controlled by nutritional intake and not growth hormones (Skuse, 1993).

- Excessive crying, frequent night waking and feeding problems in the first 4−6 months of life point to an inappropriate development of self competence of the child for internal regulation of behaviour.
- Inadequate internal behaviour regulation is reinforced and maintained by the inhibition or inadequate support of the development of internal control mechanisms of the infant.

Dysfunctional interaction of child characteristics and parental behaviour indicates a poor fit. Mother-infant interaction disturbances are thus frequently indicators of this maladaptation.

Classical and operant learning theory is only partly applicable to children in the first months of life. The newborn and small infant lacks neurological, physiological and cognitive prerequisites for the recognition of contingencies. The separation and recognition of inner and outer stimuli (cognitive abilities) and their effective qualities is only developing. For example in the first 3 months of life, withdrawal of attention (operant conditioning) when the child is crying, leads to no change in crying behaviour (e. g. Bell & Ainsworth, 1972; Hubbard & von Ijzendoorn, 1991; Meyer, Wolke, Gutbrod & Rust, submitted). The reason for this is that the infant's behaviour is biologically meaningful (i. e. to secure survival) and not learnt. However, persistent crying is maintained or reinforced by parenting behaviour that inhibits the acquisition of self-control in the infant. Examples for such inappropriate behaviour are:

- Lack of any regular routines during the day and night that support the development of behaviour regulation and predictability
- Overtiredness of the infant due to rapidly changing and over-stimulating activities

- Over-stimulation in an effort to calm the infant such as "cocktail shaker carrying", the fast and forceful rocking and shaking of the infant on the shoulder
- Under-stimulation of infants because of misperceptions about the need for sleep ("babies just eat, feed and sleep").

Parents intervene to help the infant to stop crying or to fall asleep. They, however, often inhibit or do not promote the competencies for self-soothing as no differential responses are provided, e.g. to different cry signals. For example, the mother may offer the breast at any time when the infant cries rather than using different strategies for different types of cries. Another example is that parents may always intervene immediately without giving the infant the opportunity to learn to stop crying (Demos, 1986; Larson & Aylon, 1990).

Similarly, regular organisation of the environment is necessary for the development of successful sleeping. The neurological pre-requisites for circadian sleep/wake regulation are laid at birth (Shimada et al., 1993; Wolke, 1994). The internal 'clock' has a 25 hour rhythm, that needs to be synchronised to the external 24 hour rhythm and the day and night separation needs to be established (day is for waking, night for sleeping). The most influential factors to achieve this are:

- light and darkness changes and
- regular organisation of the environment (meal times, bed times, parental intervention at sleep time).

Children have to learn to sleep through the night. While it is biologically meaningful and adaptive to wake in the first months of life for nutritional intake (Skuse at al, 1994a), this is not necessary after the first 6 months of life if the infant grows normally and the introduction to solids has taken place.

A second important bio-behavioural shift takes place at around 6−8 months when the physiological structures for effective sleep have been laid. Important cognitive changes take place that allow for an internal representation of the primary carer (e.g. separation anxiety Trevathen, 1987, Wolff, 1987, van der Maas & Hopkins, 1998). Infants in the later part of the first year develop an understanding of cause and effect and an understanding of intentions of others that start to influence the type of interactions with people (secondary inter-subjectivity). For example, infants often engage in games such as dropping a spoon, watching the spoon, looking at the mother to pick it up again, and again and again. A clear association between their action and the mother's behaviour has been made (intentional action).

- From about the 6th month of life paroxysmal crying (e.g. temper tantrums) and sleeping problems can be explained by classic and operant learning models. Crying including temper tantrums are used to reach certain goals (e.g. receiving attention). Similarly, the child cries at night to obtain attention from the parents (e.g. to be cuddled, to be taken out of the bed, to be played with at night).

Early sucking problems and vomiting are often caused by an infant's pre-disposition. Inappropriate feeding behaviour (e. g. wrong positioning, very noisy environment, changing environments) and increasing stress and anger on the side of mother further exacerbate the poor internal control of the child in dealing with food (Wolke & Skuse, 1992; Wolke, 1987; Wolke & Eldridge, 1992). Food refusal, in particular, the refusal of solid food, can be explained by a combination of biological stimuli and aversive conditioning or operant learning. Between the 4th and 6h month of life an increased sensitivity for solid food is detected. This appears to be biologically meaningful, as exclusive breastfeeding after the first 6 months of life may not be sufficient to maintain the need for calories and proteins for appropriate physical growth (Drewett et al. 1998). For example, preference for sodium that is found in only small amounts in breast milk, appears between about 3−6 months of age (Harris, 1997). In this period (4−8 months), important anatomical changes (e. g. palate) and neurological changes (biting, tongue movements etc.) lead to a general preparedness for the introduction of solid foods. If this window of opportunity is not utilised (e. g. because of prolonged exclusive breastfeeding) it becomes more difficult to introduce solid food at a later stage (Illingworth & Lister, 1964; Wolke, 1994). Infants may indicate by crying after breast or bottle feeding or night time crying, that there is a need for supplementary solid feeding (Harris, 1988; Wright, 1993). The introduction of solid foods is a delicate process occurring at a time of high nutritional requirement and represents a biologicial risk. There is a preparedness for the introduction, on the other hand infants show an inborn rejection of bitter and sour foods. They are wary of new food, which is adaptive as many sour and bitter foods in the wild are toxic. These two tendencies need to be balanced by appropriate behaviour facilitation.

- It is normal that children refuse new food occasionally. If the parents decide not to provide further solid food (continue to breast or bottle feed) or reduce the exposure to just 1 or 2 liked food products and at the same time provide a lot of attention when the child refuses food, then continuous food refusal is more likely (operant learning). If the parent show particular nervousness or strain during feeding, ("I have to get something into this child"), the unconditional stimuli anxiety and stress may be combined with the conditioned stimuli of eating which leads to an unpleasant experience and to food refusal (Lindscheid & Rasnake, 1985; see Wolke & Skuse 1992).

- Furthermore, a number of infants, who are not ready to accept solid food, may have aversive experiences when solid food is introduced. Provision of medication (aversive taste), force-feeding or over-stimulation in the oral area (e. g. using rough metal spoons) leads to an association between aversive stimuli and the food provided at the time. This is often found in infants who received oral or nasal-gastric feeding or needed oral medication (aversive conditioning; DiScipio et al., 1987).

Some have proposed that aversive conditioning is responsible for the majority of cases of food refusal. Food refusal has recently also been labelled as either food phobia, conditioned dysphagia or post-traumatic feeding disorder (Benoit and Colbear, 1998; Chatoor, Conley & Dixon, 1988). Binoit and Colbear (1998) have speculated that post-traumatic feeding disorder may become more common because of a growing number of infants are undergoing intrusive medical procedures involving mouth, nose and throat. In all cases of feeding problems eating itself is no longer associated with an enjoyable social experience or a relaxing atmosphere.

Table 3.6: Comparison of Excessive Crying-, Sleeping- and Feeding Problems: Parenting Behaviour

	Excessive Crying	Sleeping Problem	Feeding Problem
Inconsistent	*	**	**
Irregular routines	**	**	*
Maladaptive/over-stimulating	**	**	**
Inappropriate force	*	*	**
Lack of developmental support (self-control, skills)	*	**	**
Lack of positive reinforcement of other behaviours	*	*	**

It is characteristic of crying, sleeping and feeding problems that the parents use strategies to deal with an infant or toddler that are not appropriate for the developmental stage or the individual abilities of self-regulation of behaviour of the child. The caring procedures are not appropriate to support the self-regulation of the infant. Instead a complete external behavioural regulation which is not developmentally adaptive is provided by the parents, for example, the infant is breastfed, falls asleep at the breast (Wolke, 1998b), is gingerly transferred into the bed and the parents tiptoe out of the room. The child has never learnt to get to sleep and has not acquired any strategy to settle down again after waking at night. The only thing the infant can do is cry for a parent and to be fed again to fall asleep. Feeding is associated with falling asleep. Caring behaviour that maintains cry-, sleep- and feeding problems are briefly outlined in table 3.6.

3.7 Diagnosis

First, the intensity of the diagnostic process depends on whether the major symptoms are crying or sleeping problems verses feeding or growth problems. Secondly, it is important to query whether a face to face consultation is necessary or whether treatment can be done via telephone or written material. Diagnosis based on diaries and questionnaires completed by the parents and feedback via telephone conversation is a time and cost effective way of delivering primary care (Wolke et al., 1994b; Angel et al., 1990). It is thus surprising that there are so few empirical studies that have investigated whether direct contact is more successful than telephone contact. If the diagnostic information indicates complex family or psychological problems (psychiatric illness, risk of child abuse), then direct contact face to face contact is necessary. The approach which we have practised for years is based on a behavioural management strategy (Sarimski, 1993; France, 1996; Ferber and Kryger, 1995; Wolke, 1993b; 1996; 1997a for more detailed description). At the time of the initial contact (personally or via telephone) parents should always be asked how distressed they are by the child's behaviour problem. Depending on whether it is a crying or sleep problem verses a feeding problem, two different types of diagnostic strategies are pursued.

3.7.1 Excessive crying and sleeping problem

There are 2 stages in the diagnostic process:

Step 1:

- Step 1 includes a history taking of somatic problems of the child and the recording of cry, sleep and feeding behaviour of the child using a 7 day standard diary (see appendix 1).

This diary has been adapted by other groups such as Hayes (1999), Riedel-Henck, (1998) or Kast-Zahn and Morgenroth (1995). It has been validated against other parent report measures (Wolke et al., 1994b) and in comparison with recordings of crying (Barr et al., 1988). All parents should be asked whether they recently had a general paediatric investigation (e. g. by the family physician) to exclude possible organic reasons. These are rare, but occasionally crying and sleeping problems are associated with organic problems such as otitis media, infections of the urinary tract, severe oesophageal reflux, chronically enlarged tonsils etc.

For the first treatment meeting with the parents the structured assessment of the behaviour and the diary analysed.

The following information is extracted from the diary:

Crying:

- How much does the child cry?
- Is there a pattern of crying and fussing, i. e. does crying always occur at certain times during the day, is there regularity across the 7 day period?
- Is there a regular sleep and feeding pattern (i. e. is there a predictable routine for the infant)?

- How much stimulation does the child receive. Is there consistently too little or too much stimulation (e. g. play)?
- Are there strategies which are particularly effective in calming the infant?
- How does the child behave during outings, i. e. when the child visits other places?

Sleeping problems:

- How much does the child sleep at night and how many sleeping periods are there during the day?
- Is there a regular pattern of sleeping (night and day sleep, changes from bed times and waking times from day to day)?
- How long does the child take to fall asleep; where does the child fall asleep?
- How often does the child wake at night and what interventions are used?
- What do the parents do to support falling asleep?

Step 2:

- Questions are asked about the family situation, parental psycho-pathology and about the child's temperament and any other behavioural concerns.

  For this purpose parents receive 2 questionnaires (Baby and Parent questionnaire; Wolke et al., 1994b; Wolke et al., 1994d). The Baby Questionnaire includes questions about behavioural style of the child (temperament) and other problems (e. g. feeding) and the pregnancy and birth history is briefly assessed. Furthermore, parents are asked to rate how they perceive the crying of their child (e. g. painful, rejecting etc.) and what reasons they attribute to the crying or the sleeping problem of their child. How often did the parents let the child cry it out, how often did they reach the limit of their coping abilities? The Parent Questionnaire assesses demographic characteristics of the family (e. g. the living conditions and work routines, for example shift work of the father etc.) and a number of screening instruments of mental well being and disorders in the parents are included (maternal depression, partner relationship, social support systems and isolation). The living conditions and the social psychological situation of the family often determine which of the treatment suggestions can actually be put into practice by the parents.

- The information collected in step 1 and step 2 is then reviewed regarding the spectrum of problems within the family and first hypothesis are formulated about the conditions which maintain cry or sleeping problems. The probability of child abuse should be assessed, in very rare cases an admission to the clinic for some days to relieve distress may be necessary.

3.7.2 Feeding and eating problems

While the diagnosis of crying and sleeping problems and the treatment via written information and telephone contact is possible (Wolke et al., 1994b; Seymour et al.,

1989), it is not suitable for feeding problems such as food refusal, extreme food selectivity and failure to thrive. Diagnosis and treatment needs to address issues around parent-child interaction during and outside the feeding situation (e. g. play). Furthermore, a significant minority of children may have had organic reasons why they could not take in nutrition at some time, but these have already been treated. Feeding problems are often secondary to the original problems. The following diagnostic work-up may be indicated when dealing with children with food refusal (Wolke & Skuse, 1992; Skuse, Wolke & Riley 1992; Harris, 1993, Kedesdy & Budds, 1998).

3.7.2.1 Child characteristics

- All infants should receive a standard paediatric or neurological assessment as outlined by Berkowitz (1985), Frank and Zeisel (1998) or Ryder & Bithoney (1999). A full postnatal medical history is obtained, with specific enquiry about frequent infections, eczema, rashes, asthma and other allergic reactions. It is often a wise precaution to determine whether there is any degree of iron deficiency by obtaining a full blood count and serum ferritin (Schwartz, Angel & Pitcher, 1986). The physical and neurological examination, in conjunction with the history taking, should identify most chronic diseases (Goldson, 1999). Further details about specialist investigations for structural problems, oral-motor dysfunction and gastro-enterological problems are found in Krebs (1999), Reilly, Skuse and Wolke (in press) and Wolke & Skuse (1992). The determination of possible anaemia is often important, as it has physiological as well as behavioural consequences (e. g. increased infant irritability and in extreme cases apathy) and is easily treated (Auckett et al., 1986). If there is frequent vomiting, investigation for severe oesophageal reflux is indicated.
- All infants have a developmental assessment consisting of the administration of a developmental test such as the Bayley Scales of Infant Development (Bayley, 1993). This is helpful to determine whether observed interaction patterns and oral motor functioning are appropriate for the child's developmental level.
- If possible, oral-motor functioning using a standard procedure such as the Schedule for Oral Motor Assessment (SOMA, Reilly et al. 1995; in press; Mathisen et al., 1989) should be carried out. In this assessment, the infant is presented with different types and textures of food, and oral motor behaviours are filmed in close up. The assessment also includes an examination for oral hyper-sensitivity to touch and for any structural problems in the intra-oral area, such as high arch palate in which food may be impacted (Reilly et al., 1995).
- The behaviour of the infant is assessed via questionnaires completed by the parents, via ratings of behaviour during developmental testing (Tester's Rating of Infant Behaviour; Wolke, Skuse & Mathisen, 1990a). These ratings provide infor-

mation on how the infant behaves with a stranger and whether behavioural problems are specific to the feeding situation or are pervasive.

- A mealtime is video taped. It is preferable that this is done at home where the child normally eats. If a home visit is not possible, parents can be given a video camera to film mealtimes at home.

Furthermore, interactions in a structured play situation should be filmed to assess whether the interaction problems which may be present during feeds are specific to eating or generalised (see Feeding Interaction Scale, Wolke 1986a, Play Observation Scheme and Emotion Rating; Wolke, 1986b; recent investigations: Skuse et al., 1992; Wolke et al., 1990, Stein et al; 1993; Lindberg, 1994; Lindberg et al., 1996).

- The parents should complete a 7-day dietary diary or a food frequency questionnaire (for some parents a diary is too demanding and a food frequency questionnaire may be sufficient).

There are various computer programmes which allow analysis of the nutritional diaries to be analysed by a dietician according to calorie, protein and fat intake. The diary may give some indication for under-nutrition. The food frequency questionnaire provides information regarding the variety of foods offered to the child.

- A short screening for psychiatric problems (e. g. depression or anxiety) should be carried out (see section on crying and sleeping problems).
- The height and weight of both parents and the index child's siblings should be determined. Berkowitz (1980) reported that 15% of parents of infants seen in her feeding clinic have " constitutional" short stature. We are cautious of drawing the conclusion that infants may be growing poorly because their parents are relatively small. These parents may have suffered growth failure in their own childhood because of environmental deprivation.

3.8 Treatment of crying and sleeping problems

Step 3:

After all diagnostic information has been collected the hypotheses are discussed with the parents and the treatment is jointly planned with them.

In the first treatment session the experience of the parents with their diary is discussed. Parents are treated as *competent partners* in the treatment. They have often gained an accurate picture about the type and severity of the problem, and formulated their own hypotheses of what may have led to the crying or sleeping problem. The therapist suggests a number of hypotheses and probes whether the parents agree or reject specific hypotheses. There are often more than one problem, and it is important to build a hierarchy of problems:

- Identify the first and most important problem for the parents. This problem be-haviour should be treatable within 2 weeks.
- Derive a therapy contract and inform the parents that interventions that are carried out inconsistently often increase rather than reduce the problem. Warn the parents that changes in caring behaviour are often necessary which can be stressful at the beginning. If the suggestions are not acceptable to the parents, it is often better not to even try them. Discuss alternative management principles.
- Consequences of any therapy success should be discussed. Crying and sleeping problems are often problems one can talk about with other mothers which facili-tates social contacts. A therapy success could mean a loss of these opportunities. Or a child that is sleeping between husband and wife may provide a buffer against intimate contacts between the parents. It should be pointed out to the parents that a child should never be used for problems which the parents may have!

Concrete strategies are chosen according to the following principles:

- The therapy is individualised for each family
- It is appropriate for the developmental level of the child
- It supports the development of internal behaviour control of the child, this means that the child will be helped to calm down or to fall asleep alone

3.8.1 Intervention strategies for young infants (less than 6 months old)

The major aim of these interventions is to create adaptive environmental conditions to improve internal behavioural control. These suggestions are of interest for the *prevention* of crying and sleeping problems:

- Provide the parents with information about the normal development of crying and sleeping. Explain that there is large variation between infants so that parents can develop realistic expectations.
- Infants who have poor self-control require increased regularity in their daily life. This should include strict times for feeding, sleeping, playing, outings etc. The differences in parental behaviour between day and night time should be maxi-mised (at night time only feeding for nutritional purposes, no eye contact, no lights on and no talking while feeding). This will provide a predictability of events for the infant.
- Over-stimulation (frequent carrying, swaddling, persistent talking to the infant, changing stimuli in quick succession etc.) should be reduced. The child is not calm and has no chance to calm down. These infants are often over tired and react with irritability to the high level of stimulation.
- Parents should learn to observe their baby. Many parents who have got a crying baby or an infant who doesn't sleep at night are attuned to fussing and crying behaviour (negative behaviour of the child). When the child stops crying or falls

asleep (positive behaviour), this behaviour is often ignored. These periods are used to recover from the long periods of negative behaviour. It is important that the parents re-learn to focus on positive behaviour and to react to the infant with increased attention and positive expression during positive behaviour periods (re-inforcement).

- Methods that prevent the child learning to initiate behaviour control should be avoided. These are tricks parents often use to get their child to sleep. Examples are:
  car rides to get the infant to sleep, feeding until the child is asleep, or the parents let the child fall asleep on the couch in front of the television.
- Clear association between environmental cues and sleeping should be built up. At night, the infant should always fall asleep in the same place (for example, in the own crib or bed). Walking or providing a dummy is perfectly permissible, but the infant should not use the dummy or being rocked until s/he has completely fallen asleep.
- The baby should always fall asleep with the secure feeling that the parents are close by.
- Stimulating play an hour before it is time to go to bed is not advisable. Often when the father or mother return home after a day's work they want to use the last hour before bedtime as "quality time". This is often filled with stimulating games including rocking, throwing the child into the air and in older children talking about the day. It is difficult for a small child to be highly stimulated at one moment and to be expected to fall asleep the next!
- Some mothers discontinue breastfeeding because night wakings are too distressing. The longest period of night time sleep can be stretched by the use of focal feeds. The infant is put to bed at a reasonable time (e.g. 8 pm) and is awoken when the mother goes to bed (e.g. between 11 pm−midnight). This way the mother takes control over the feeding process and secondly the periods until the next feed during the night (after 5 am) are subsequently stretched. The success of this procedure has been described by Pinnilla and Birch (1993).
- Sensitivity to crying does not mean that the parents react immediately to every fuss. There are no rules how long one should wait, rather the parents should react according to the situation (hunger-cry, pain-cry versus bored cry). Waiting for up to 2 minutes is appropriate in some circumstances to allow the infant to calm down. Parents of cry babies have often lost their intuitive "checking" of different causes of crying and react very quickly, agitated and use a variety of over-stimulating interventions.

3.8.2 Intervention strategies for children over 6 months of age

A wide variety of behavioural methods such as extinction and their modifications (checking, time out) as well as shaping (graded approaches) are applicable for this age group (Douglas & Richman, 1984).

- The child has to be tired when it is asked to fall asleep. The longest sleep period follows the longest period of waking. Most children with night waking problems have irregular sleep rhythm, i. e. they partly compensate night waking by sleeping during the day. Many children with night waking problems are over-tired and irritable and more difficult during the day (Minde et al., 1994). The parents are often happy when their infant or toddler sleeps at least for a few hours during the day. This, however, maintains inappropriate sleeping patterns. Parents have to take control over the child's sleep rhythm:
- Regularity in daily routines regarding eating, playing and bed times need to be built up.
- Bed times need to be placed at an appropriate time for infant and according to the life style of the parents, usually between 7 and 9 pm.
- The daily sleep needs to be regulated, e. g. a child who has slept between 4 and 6 pm is usually not prepared to go to sleep at 8 o'clock (there are exceptions). In these cases the child should not be allowed to sleep after 3.30 pm in the afternoon. Any infant should not sleep more than 4 hours in one stretch during the day to compensate for night waking.
- The child should have a fulfilling day. The day should include physical activities and playing outdoors which tires the child.
- Clear evening and settling routines need to be established (Wolke, 1998b). Falling asleep and night waking problems are closely related to each other: Infants and toddlers who have not learnt to fall asleep by themselves have not learnt any strategy to soothe themselves once they wake up at night. They can only cry, call or go to their parents (Mindell and Durand, 1993; Wolke et al., 1994a; Wolke, 1997b, c).
- Clearly defined rituals which provide security for the child should be carried out every night. Such a sequence could look as follows: the child is asked to go to their room, to change into pyjamas, wash or have a bath, brush their teeth, joint looking at picture book in the child's room, then to put the child into bed to fall asleep. Many children with sleeping problems react with crying or shouting when the parents leave the room in the evening. Appropriate behaviour can be built up using a *graded approach,* often called *shaping.*
- A parent stays with the child in the first night until it is just about falling asleep. The parent then leaves the room and returns the first night after 2 minutes, the second night after 5 minutes, the third night after 10 minutes etc. to the child. At these times they may reassure the child, but not pick them up or cuddle them and never stay until the child is completely asleep.

This is a graded extinction approach which does not leave the child to cry it out, rather the parents come back, but do not use any reinforcement such as holding, stroking, taking the child out of bed or additional attention.

- No over-stimulation: Any stimulating and arousing games are forbidden 1 hour before going to sleep.

It is often the mothers who have to deal with the child waking at night. On the one hand this makes them very tired, but on the other hand they are worried about leaving their child alone. It is difficult for some mothers to impose clear rules at bed time because they find it difficult to let go of the child or feel compassion for the child.

- It is thus often important that fathers should be involved in the therapy right from the beginning. Fathers should be allowed to deal with the child at bedtime and establish a clear bed time routine (Minde et al., 1993). Important is that the mother doesn't interfere when the child cries, which often occurs when new bed time routines are introduced. We have previously asked the mother to leave the house at bedtime and to visit a friend. This makes it easier for the father to carry out the full bedtime routine.

These management suggestions not only alleviate falling asleep problems, but also often dramatically improve night sleeping (Mindell & Durand, 1993). If these changes in settling the child do not improve night time sleeping there is a wide repertoire of behaviour modification techniques (Wolke, 1997c).

- Extinction:
  when the child cries at night it is left to cry it out. This is usually very successful but is not accepted by most parents and should not be tried if the parents can't implement it (Rickett & Johnson, 1988; France, 1994). It is also not appropriate for small children who make themselves vomit or use excessive head banging to attract the parents' attention.
- Checking is as described above, a modified version of extension by parents providing a short verbal reassurance to the child ("Mum & Dad are here, don't worry, go back to sleep") and other reinforcers (physical contact, taking child into parental bed, games at night etc.) are withdrawn. It is important that parents apply the checking procedure consistently, as any intermittent reinforcement due to regression back to old behavioural patterns weakens any newly built up associations. It is important to inform the parents that a child, that has positive and loving interactions with their parents during the day does not suffer from the checking procedure. Application of checking together with the other suggestions for falling asleep and daily rhythms lead to sleeping through the night in most children within 2 weeks (Ferber, 1987; Richman et al. 1985).
- If a toddler wakes regularly at the same time during the night, e.g. at 11 pm, 2 am and 4 am, a parent controlled schedule to waken the child can be applied. The parents take control for night waking by waking the child always a quarter of an hour before it would normally wake. The association between self-initiated waking of the child and reinforcement (parents will come) is broken, the child loses the control. This method is used for parents who cannot accomplish the checking method and it is usually successful, but will take about twice as long as the checking procedure to eliminate night waking (Rickett & Johnson, 1988).

It is important that parent characteristics, partner support and environmental conditions (living situation) are considered when making treatment suggestions. The parents need to be prepared that some procedures such as checking will lead to an initial increase in inadequate behaviour (e. g. crying) but that this will reduce over the subsequent nights.

What has been taken during the night, needs to be given during the day. Parents have to be made aware that it is important to show the child how much it is loved and accepted.

Wolke (1999) has described a number of day-time actions that help to make the child feel loved.

- Observe your child, be there with your full attention
- Listen to your child, repeat what they say to enhance communication
- Always label the action and not the child
- Use short instructions and provide positive feedback. Apologise if you have done something wrong. The child learns that their feelings count
- Be a positive model for your child
- Give clear instructions that your child can understand what you want
- Encourage role play
- Provide physical reinforcement using verbal and physical contact mode rather than sweet or material objects

3.9 Treatment of feeding and eating problems

The diagnostic information from observation, history taking and oral motor assessment are reviewed. As with crying and sleeping problems, intervention needs to be tailored to the family's needs and resources. The decision to proceed with any treatment for feeding problems should rest on answering the following questions (Kedesdy & Budd, 1998):

1. Is feeding intervention necessary for medical reasons? What will happen in the longer term if no intervention is initiated?
2. Are the caregivers receptive to environmental intervention at the present time?
3. Are sufficient resources available to support the family and implement the intervention with a reasonable chance of success?

If the consequences for the child are severe (e. g. severe under-nutrition or risk of abuse and severe family problems) then an intervention is indicated independent of the answers to question 2 and 3. However, the success will depend on the motivation of the parents and the readiness for intervention and the resources available to carry out the intervention and this needs to be discussed with the parents and written into the therapy contract.

3.9.1 Food refusers

As an example, a therapeutic approach for food refusal problems is briefly outlined (see Wolke & Skuse, 1992 for a more detailed account of treatment and see table 7 – Behavioural management techniques);

- Provide the right environmental conditions for meal times. Food refusers are often more sensitive to environmental distractions. It is thus important that the environment is arranged in such a way that it doesn't distract from eating (no radio/television, no other people who are not eating themselves). The utensils should be appropriate for the child, e. g. plastic rather than metal spoons should be used. A full list of feeding intervention parameters is to be found in Wolke & Skuse (1992). To facilitate some nutritional intake, parents often adopt feeding positions which are inadequate for the developmental status of the child (e. g. feeding a 10 months old lying on the mother's lap). In these circumstances adequate positioning in the high chair with good side support and foot support allowing the child to sit in the upright position to support swallowing, is recommended.
- Foods of different tastes should be offered at each meal time (exposure) and the food should be made available to the child to experiment with.
  Sometimes a mother removes the food from the child's reach so that the infant doesn't play around and doesn't make a mess. Many food refusers have had aversive experience with certain foods and food itself has become an aversive stimuli. In those situations, exploration by the child of the food (e. g. touching) should be encouraged. Some children reject any type of food, others reject solid food, i. e. they accept mash or drinks. Many of the children with food refusal have a restricted selection of food. New acceptance of food is built up by *exposure*. The child is given food with new tastes at each meal. This can be facilitated by applying this new food to the lips of the child. The initial aim is that the child explores the new tastes and consistencies (e. g. solid food). Furthermore, graded approaches are used to introduce solid food. The thin purée gets thickened from day to day until small solid pieces can be introduced.
- Behaviour and oral motor problems of children can be treated by behaviour therapeutic methods. Behavioural intervention procedures are rooted in learning theory and can be applied to socially relevant problems to strengthen adaptive behaviours and to reduce maladaptive behaviours. Of particular interest in clinical feeding interventions are: aspects of the feeders' responses that have an inadvertent impact on feeding patterns (e. g. food refusal and only offering limited preferred food by parent) and also) techniques for "unlearning" or modifying maladaptive feeding patterns (e. g. spitting out food and receiving a lot of attention by parents) by re-arranging social and environmental concomitance to feeding (Kedesdy & Budd, 1998; Wolke, Skuse & Reilly, in press; Reilly et al., 1995; Tuchman & Walter, 1994). There are a range of adapted techniques that can be

used in infants from 6 months of age onwards. An overview of the behaviour intervention strategies are given in table 5. It is important to point out that the techniques outlined in table 5 are usually effective as part of an individualised package of strategies that parents can apply. Some of the individual techniques may not be acceptable to some parents. Important other ingredients of treatment programmes include parental modelling, changes in the physical and social feeding environment, exposure to different tastes and textures and emotional support of the parents. For a detailed discussion of the application of these techniques for feeding problems, see Wolke et al. (in press).

- A relaxed parent-child interaction should be created. In rare cases, the feeding disorder is a result of severe maternal psychopathology (e. g. major depression, psychosis, severe learning disability or eating disorder of the mother). In these cases the child will often eat normally with other people. More often, problems that the mother experiences are a reaction to the feeding problems (self-doubt, depressive symptoms, anxiety etc.). The behaviour of these mothers is often not adaptive and variable ranging from "laissez faire" to force feeding (Lindberg et al., 1996). The parental behaviour towards the child during meal times becomes completely fixated on nutritional intake. Fun and play during the feeding situation has been completely lost (Wolke & Skuse, 1992). The parents concentrate on the difficult behaviour of the child (e. g. food rejection, spitting out) and ignore the social behaviour during meals. Often the mothers become very nervous during mealtimes, consistently offer food and try to trick the child to accept some food (e. g. they show a toy and when the child smiles at the toy they quickly insert a spoon into the mouth and forcefully close the mouth to force swallowing of the food). "To get food into the child" and constant control of weight gain *should not be the primary goal at the beginning of treatment* aiming at improving mother-child interaction. Unfortunately, paediatricians and other health professionals often provide advice that increases anxiety in mothers (weighing before and after feeds, weighing of the child at every visit to the practice).

The central focus of the therapy is to make eating a pleasurable experience again (Black & Teti, 1997). Neither weighing nor nutritional intake is of importance at the beginning of the intervention. The child has not gained weight for months despite all the efforts of the mother during meal times. Meal times should be video-taped once or twice per week and the therapist reviews the video tape and marks particularly positive versus negative reactions of the child. These selected sequences are played back to the mother and she is asked to interpret and provide explanations for the child's behaviour and hers (Wolke & Skuse, 1992). The mother is treated as a *competent co-therapist* and not bombarded with advice. Where positive reactions of the child are found, the behaviour of the mother is reinforced and strategies are discussed of how the mother can build on the behaviour shown. When negative reactions are found, alternative behaviour is discussed that would be acceptable to

Table 3.7: Overview of behaviour management principles and applications to feeding interventions

Underlying principle	Description of application	Examples
To increase desired behaviours		
Positive reinforcement	Provide positive consequences for desired behaviour	Give praise, physical affection, or tangible rewards (tokens).
Negative reinforcement	Terminate aversive stimulus contingent on desired behaviour	Release physical restraint (for food expulsion) when child accepts food.
Discrimination	Reinforce target behaviour in presence of defined stimulus.	Praise modelled behaviour of eating. Reward cooperation with feeding requests.
Shaping	Reinforce successive approximations toward desired response.	Praise 1) looking at food, then 2) allowing food to touch lips, then 3) opening mouth, then 4) accepting food.
Fading	Gradually remove assistance and reinforcement needed to maintain behaviour.	Decrease extent of guidance and rewards as child gains self-feeding skills.
Exposure/Flooding (stimulus-response)	Provide food stimuli to reduce aversion	expose to different tastes and textures (e. g. applied to toys)
To decrease undesired behaviours		
Extinction	Withhold rewarding stimulus contingent on target response	Ignore mild inappropriate behaviour. Continue prompts during escape behaviour.
Satiation	Continually present desired stimulus until it loses its reinforcing value.	Offer unlimited portions of food to reduce rumination.
Punishment	Present aversive stimulus or remove rewarding stimulus contingent on undesired behaviour	Use time-out. Give verbal reprimand. Restrict toys. Use overcorrection.
Desensitization	Pair conditioned aversive stimulus with absence of aversive events or with present of positive events.	Distract child during fearful procedure. Use gentle massage to promote acceptance of touch.

Source: Kedesdy and Budd, 1998.

the mother. The discussion is summarised and a list of alternatives is drawn up at the end of the session and handed to the parents. It is often the case that during the first few days working with food refusers that no or little nutrition is actively inserted. The child relearns to play with the spoon, the food bowl and food. Any approach of the child, for example, touching the mouth with the food, licking food of the fingers etc. is positively reinforced by special attention given by the mother (shaping) and any rejection is ignored. Our and other studies (Skuse et al., 1992; Lindberg et al., 1996) indicate that food refusers often indicate what they do not like. In contrast, they are poor in communicating what they would like. Thus highly sensitive perception of small nuances need to be trained.

- Changes in the household organisation: the child has to be hungry. Families who experience other social stress or have a high professional workload often lack a clear and regular meal time plan. Eating occurs standing up or in front of the television, the timing of meal times varies largely or there is continuous "snacking". For example, we observed in one family who travelled between three different apartments and worked in the media industry, that the daughter did not receive any food for up to 18 hours as she did not indicate any demand for food. *Lack of hunger feeling* and lack of communicating demand for food is a frequent observation in feeding problem children.

It is thus important that a clear daily routine of meal times is established. No snacks are allowed between meal times. Fast food should be avoided and a home prepared diet should be offered. Recipes can be provided by dieticians. Joint meal times with all family members should take place at least once during the day. Other children and the parents can be a model for good eating (Satter, 1995). In older pre-school children, eating together with other children (for example in the nursery, in the hospital) provides an important model for the establishment of food acceptance (Birch, 1980).

- All treatments, whether for crying, sleeping or feeding problems should be followed up 3 months after the parents have been discharged from care for these problems.

3.10 Empirical evaluation of treatment methods

There are 3 major approaches for the treatment of excessive crying and sleeping problems. These include pharmacological therapy (e. g. Hwang & Danielson, 1985; Simonoff & Stores, 1987; Dahl, 1992), dietary changes (e. g. Kahn et al., 1989, Hill & Hoskin, 1995) and a range of behavioural management approaches (Wolke, 1993b; Wolke et al. 1994b). A fourth approach is the use of psychodynamic treatment of the mother-infant relationship (e. g. Daws, 1985); and finally the use of naturopathic interventions such as herbal teas (Weizman et al., 1993) has been recently proposed.

Results of studies regarding the treatment of excessive crying have been recently reviewed by Wolke (1993b; 1997a; Wolke et al. (1994b), Wolke and Meyer (1995) and Lucassen et al. (1998). There is agreement across the systematic reviews that pharmacological treatment for excessive crying (e. g. simethicone, dicyclomine) (e. g.

Lucassen et al., 1998) or sleeping problems (e. g. Richman et al., 1985b) may lead to a reduction of symptoms but leads to no long term remediation of problems. Furthermore, dicyclomine has been withdrawn from the market as a colic treatment due to a number of possible deaths associated with the treatment in young infants (Williams & Watkins-Jones, 1984). Dietary treatments including changes in diets of breastfeeding mothers, soy formula or hypoallergenic formulations or low lactose formulations for formula fed infants have been found to show some significant effect (Lucassen et al., 1998). However, as argued by Wolke & Meyer (1995) or Forsyth, 1989) these trials were often conducted with selected populations who had been referred for treatment to gastroenterologists because of a high loading of atopic problems in the families. It has been estimated that only a minority of about 5– 10% of infants with either crying or sleeping problems (Kahn et al., 1989; Wolke, 1993b) will benefit from dietary treatment. Furthermore, the effects of e. g. cow milk protein intolerance may be short lived in early infancy and should not suggest a long term vulnerability (Forsyth & Canny, 1993; Wolke & Meyer, 1995).

A variety of behavioural approaches have received empirical evaluation. However, behavioural studies cannot be judged according to the same criteria as dietary or drug trials as they often cannot be double blind and the use of randomisation is often difficult (e. g. waiting control groups) due to high subject loss or ethical considerations. Simple behavioural approaches have included increased carrying (e. g. Barr et al., 1991) in baby carriers, car ride simulators (e. g. SleepTight TM, Parkin et al., 1993) or baby-massage (Elliott & Reilly, 1998). None of these "easy recipe" approaches showed no advantages compared to controls for the treatment of excessive crying. In contrast, studies that employed treatment by changing parent behaviour such as reducing stimulation (McKenzie, 1991) or multiple parenting strategies to manage infant crying (e. g. as outlined here; Wolke et al., 1994b) showed that behavioural management is successful in reducing excessive crying (see Wolke, 1993b, 1997b for a review). However, a randomised controlled trial fulfilling all necessary criteria for a "perfect" treatment trial is still outstanding due to often strong ethical and practical constraints.

A systematic review of empirical behavioural studies of sleeping problems are to be found in table 3.8. The majority of studies employed a pre- to post-test design, i. e. the changes in symptoms were evaluated before and after the treatment. This is sufficient for clinical documentation, but decisive studies require appropriate non-treatment control groups. Many children with less severe sleeping problems show spontaneous remission and a pre- to post-treatment design is unable to inform about the relative frequency of this group (see Wolke et al., 1994b). All sleeping problem studies reported improvements, however, only 5 of 12 studies indicated significant improvement in more than 75% of cases (s. Tab. 3.8).

The psychodynamic treatment of the mother-child relationship (Daws, 1985; Robert-Tissot et al., 1996; 1998) focuses mainly on the interpersonal and affective relation-

Table 3.8: Summary of treatment studies of sleeping problems

Study	Age in Months	N of Interv Group	Length of Interv in Wks	% Impve	Cf Slp Diff Control	Night waking N/W or N/D^
General Behavioral Management						
Sanger at al. (1981)	7–60	16	~3	56	–	–
Weir & Dinnick (1988)	4–54	21		59	n.s.	–
Seymour et al. (1983)	<72	208	~5	78	–	NW 6.6 > 1.6*
Jones & Verduyn (1983)		19	~4	53	–	?
Richman et al. (1985)	12–60	35	24	90	-	?
Seymour et al. (1989)	9–60	15			signif.	W/N 2.3 > 1*
Messer et al. (1994)	13	23	4	60	n.s.	W/N 2.2 > 1.8*
Minde et al. (1993)/ Minde (1994)	28	12–36	~8	83	–	–
Bramble (1997)	3–12 LD	15	2	80	–	–
Extinction						
Rickert & Johnson (1988)	6–54	11	8	–	signif.	W/N 1 > 0.3*
France (1992)	6–24	35	6	–	signif.	–
Checking						
Sadeh (1994)	9–24	25	1–3	60	–	W/N 3.7 > 1.6*
Graduated Extinction						
Mindell & Durand (1993)	18–52	6	1	100	–	W/N 1.5 > 0.2*

~ approximately
^ N/W number of nights woken/week W/N number of wakings per night
* significant reduction in wakings

ship of the mother with her infant. However, apart from the study by Robert-Tissot et al. (1996) there is a lack of any systematic evaluation of this approach. Furthermore, many behavioural techniques are often integrated in this approach (e. g. Daws, 1985). The psychodynamic contribution emphasising the importance of the affective relationship is important to recognise as "pure" behavioural approaches that ignore the dynamic of the family and mother-infant interaction are often not implemented or ignore important factors maintaining crying or sleeping problems. There is still a need for controlled studies that investigate different treatment approaches, compare different consultation types (written, telephone, face-to-face) and are systematically evaluated regarding cost-effectiveness (see Wolke & Schulz, 1999).

Controlled studies concerned with the treatment of severe feeding problems are generally lacking. However, there are a range of publications on case series or single case studies that evaluated different types of mostly behavioural approaches (e. g. Linscheid & Rasnake, 1985; DiScipio, et al., 1978; Hanks et al., 1988; Iwaniec et al., 1985; Wolke & Skuse, 1992; Harris, 1993; Kedesky & Budd, 1998; Satter, 1995; Duniz et al., 1996; Werle et al., 1993; Shore et al., 1998; Benoit & Colbear, 1998). The treatments are usually eclectic integrating a number of behavioural methods. The case series indicate that behavioural approaches are very successful in dealing with severe feeding problems although proper efficacy studies are indicated. Three controlled studies have been conducted with failure to thrive (FTT) infants in affluent societies. Two were conducted on clinic populations (Drotar & Sturm, 1988; Haynes et al., 1984) and one employed regular home visits with the aim of altering family interactions and caring behaviour. Haynes et al. (1984) found that the clinic intervention had no positive effects on either growth, cognitive development or mother-infant interaction after 6 months. Drotar & Sturm (1988) also found no improvements of regular home visits on the cognitive development of infants showing a failure to thrive at 3 years of age. Black et al. (1995) reported on the only randomised clinical trial of home intervention for children with failure to thrive in the community. 116 mothers participated split in two groups (home visits vs. standard paediatric care). Those in the home intervention group had on average 19 visits by trained lay visitors. The results have been disappointing. All children independent of group showed small improvement in weight for age while the developmental quotients and language scores showed a downfall during the observation period although interaction quality improved slightly in both groups. These findings indicate that FTT and severe feeding problems are generally difficult to treat and persistent problems. A criticism of the Black et al. (1995) is that the home visiting did not focus specifically on eating but assumed that FTT is due to general parenting problems, which has not been confirmed in large community studies (Wolke, 1996). Unspecific programmes not developed for certain problem groups are often unsuccessful as has been shown in other fields (Wolke, 1991; Wolke & Schulz, 1999). In contrast, preventive strategies that promote specific interaction during feeding appear to be successful. Black & Teti (1997) showed that a video about effective feeding of the infant shown to adolescent mothers can change attitudes and to a lesser extent the behaviour of adolescent mothers.

Regarding the treatment of regulatory disturbances, i. e. infants with multiple behavioural problems case reports are available (e. g. v. Hofacker & Papousek, 1998). While this study audits the treatment and indicates differences to infants without regulatory problems, there are no systematic controlled intervention studies that have systematically evaluated the use of a complex system approach for treatment of regulatory disturbance.

3.11 Summary and conclusions

Excessive crying, sleeping and feeding problems in infants can be considered as *disturbances of regulation and integration* of biological and social functioning. Crying, sleeping and feeding have primary biological functions and the aetiological factors and methods of treatment differ according to developmental *age* (i. e. before vs. after 6 months of age). There are a variety of treatment approaches. While dietary treatment may be highly successful for a minority of crying and sleep problem children, behavioural management has been shown to help a large number of infants and their parents in managing with early crying, sleeping and feeding problems.

There are a number of questions that require to be addressed in further clinical research: (a) Can children with significant co-morbidity be considered as a separate regulatory disturbed group of children? (b) What components of treatment are most effective and efficient in clinical practice? Further efficacy and efficiency studies are necessary (Wolke & Schulz, 1999). (c) What new innovative media can be used for preventive strategies? These may include the use of the internet for diagnosis and advice, written information, counselling via telephone or via video link. These methods are most relevant in primary care and can utilise resources such as trained lay-counsellors (e. g. Wolke et al., 1994b). Costly multi-modal treatment is more appropriate for severe feeding problems or where there are psychological problems of the parents or a high risk of child abuse.

3.12 Literature

[1] American Academy of Pediatrics (1993). Shaken Baby Syndrome: inflicted cerebral trauma. Pediatrics, 92, 872–875.

[2] American Academy of Pediatrics, Committee on Nutrition (1989). Hypoallergenic infant formulas. Pediatrics, 83 (6), 1068–1069.

[3] Anders TF (1994). Infant sleep, night-time relationships, and attachment. Psychiatry, 57, 11–21.

[4] Angel, S., Nicoll, J., & Amatiello, W. (1990). Assessing the need for an out-of-hours telephone advisory service. Health Visitor, 63 (7), 225–227.

[5] Atkinson, E., Vetere, A., & Grayson, K. (1995). Sleep disruption in young children. The influence of temperament on the sleep patterns of pre-school children. Child: Care, Health and Development, 21, 233–246.

[6] Auckett, M. A., Parks, Y. A., Scott, P. H., & Wharton, B. A. (1986). Treatment with iron increases weight gain and psychomotor development. Archives of Disease in Childhood, 61, 849–857.

[7] Barr, R. G. (1990). The normal crying curve: what do we really know? Developmental Medicine and Child Neurology, 32, 356–362.
Barr, R. G. (in press). Excessive crying. In M. Lewis & A. Sameroff (Eds.), Handbook of Developmental Psychopathology (2 ed.,).

[8] Barr, R. G., Chen, S., Hopkins, B., & Westra, T. (1996). Crying patterns in preterm infants. Developmental Medicine and Child Neurology, 38, 345–355.

[9] Barr, R. G., McMullan, S. J., Spiess, H., Leduc, D. G., Yaremko, J., Barfield, R., Francoeur, E., & Hunziker, U. A. (1991). Carrying as colic "therapy": a randomised controlled trial. Pediatrics, 87, 623–630.

[10] Bates, J. E., Viken, R. J., Alexander, D., Beyers, J., & Stockton, L. (1995,). Sleep and adjustment in preschool children. Paper presented at the Meeting of Society for Research in Child Development, Indianapolis.

[11] Bayley, N. (1993). Bayley Scales of Infant Development- Second Edition, Assessment focus – people products quality. The Psychological Corporation, Order Service Centre, P.O. Box 839954, San Antonio, TX 78283–3954.

[12] Bell, S. M., & Ainsworth, D. S. (1972). Infant crying and maternal responsiveness. Child Development, 43, 1171–1190.

[13] Benoit, D., Zeanah, C. H., Boucher, C., & Minde, K. K. (1992). Sleep disorders in early childhood: association with insecure maternal attachment. Journal of American Academic Child and Adolescent Psychiatry, 31 (1), 86–92.

[14] Birch, L. L. (1980). Effects of peer models' food choices and eating behaviours on pre-schoolers' food preferences. Child Development, 51, 489–496.

[15] Black, M. M., Dubowitz, H., Hutchson, J., Berenson-Howard, J., & Starr, J. H. (1995). A randomised clinical trial of home intervention for children with failure to thrive. Pediatrics, 95, 807–814.

[16] Black, M. M., & Teti, L. O. (1997). Promoting mealtime communication between adolescent mothers and their infants through videotape. Pediatrics, 99, 432–437.

[17] Blurton-Jones, N., Rossetti-Ferreira, M. C., Farquar-Brown, M., & Macdonald, L. (1978). The association between perinatal factors and later night waking. Developmental Medicine and Child Neurology, 20, 427–434.

[18] Boddy, J. M. (1997). Maternal characteristics and development of children who failed to thrive. Unpublished Ph.D. thesis, University of London, London.

[19] Bramble, D. (1997). Rapid-acting treatment for a common sleep problem. Dev Med Child Neurol, 39 (8), 543–547.

[20] Brandt, I. (1983). Griffiths Entwicklungsskalen (GES zur Beurteilung der Entwicklung in den ersten beiden Lebensjahren). Weinheim: Beltz.

[21] Burnham, M. M., Anders, T. F., Gaylor, E. E., & Goodlin-Jones, B. L. (1998, 2–5 April). Night-to-night consistency of sleep variables over the first year: A preliminary analysis. Paper presented at the International Conference for Infant Studies, Atlanta.

[22] Carey, W. B. (1985). Temperament and increased weight gain in infants. Developmental and Behavioral Pediatrics, 6 (3), 128–131.

[23] Carey, W. B. (1990). Infantile colic: a paediatric practitioner-researcher's point of view. Infant Mental Health Journal, 11, 334–339.

[24] Dahl, M., Rydell, A. M., & Sundelin, C. (1994). Children with early food refusal to eat. Acta Paediatrica, 83, 54–58.

[25] Dahl, M., & Sundelin, C. (1986). Early feeding problems in an affluent society: Categories and clinical signs. Acta Paediatrica Scandinavica, 75, 370–375.

[26] Dahl, M., & Kristiansson, B. (1987). Early feeding problems in an affluent society. IV. Impact on growth up to two years of age. Acta Paediatrica Scandinavica, 76, 881–888.

[27] Dahl, M., & Sundelin, C. (1992). Feeding problems in an affluent society. Follow-up at four years of age. Acta Paediatrica, 81, 575–579.

[28] Dahl, R. E. (1992). The pharmacologic treatment of sleep disorders. Psychiatric Clinics of North America, 15 (1), 161–178.

[29] Daws, D. (1985). Through the Night: Helping parents and sleepless infants. London: Free Association Books.

[30] DeGangi, G. A., DiPietro, J. A., Greenspan, S. I., & Porges, S. (1991). Psycho-physiological characteristics of the regulatory disordered infant. Infant Behaviour and Development, 14, 37–50.

[31] Demos, V. (1986). Crying in early infancy: an illustration of the motivational function of affect. In T. B. Brazelton & M. Yogman (Eds.), Affective Development in Infancy (pp. 122–156). Norwood, NJ: Ablex.

[32] Di Scipio, W. J., Kaslon, K., & Ruben, R. J. (1978). Traumatically acquired conditioned dysphagia in children. Annals of Otology, 87, 509–514.

[33] Douglas, J., & Richman, N. (1984). My child won't sleep. Harmondsworth, Middlesex: Penguin Books.

[34] Dowdney, L., Skuse, D., Heptinstall, E., Puckering, C., & Zur-Szpiro, S. (1987). Growth retardation and developmental delay amongst inner-city children. Journal of Child Psychology and Psychiatry., 28 (4), 529–541.

[35] Dowdney, L., Skuse, D., Morris, K., & Pickles, A. (in press). Short normal children and environmental disadvantage: a longitudinal study of growth and cognitive development from 4 to 11 years. Journal of Child Psychology and Psychiatry.

[36] Drewett, R., Wright, P., & Young, B. (1998). From feeds to meals: The development of hunger and food intake in infants and young children. In C. A. Niven & A. Walker (Eds.), Current issues in infancy and parenthood (Vol. 3, pp. 204–217). Oxford: Butterworth-Heinemann.

[37] Drewett, R. E., Corbett, S. S., & Wright, C. M. (in press). Cognitive and educational attainments at school age of children who failed to thrive in infancy: a population based study. Journal of Child Psychology and Psychiatry.

[38] Drotar, D., & Sturm, L. (1988). Prediction of intellectual development in young children with histories of non-organic failure to thrive. Journal of Pediatric Psychology, 13, 281–296.

[39] Duniz, M., Scheer, P. J., Trojovsky, A., Kaschnitz, W., Kvas, E., & Macari, S. (1996). Changes in psychopathology of parents of NOFT (non-organic failure to thrive) infants during treatment. European Child and Adolescent Psychiatry, 5, 93–100.

[40] Elliott, R. M., & Reilly, S. M. (1998, 2–5 April). Effect of selected soothing techniques of parent-infant interaction and on infant crying. Paper presented at the 11th International Conference of Infant Studies, Atlanta, USA.

[41] Ferber, R. (1987). The sleepless child. In C. Guilleminault (Ed.), Sleep and its disorders in children (pp. 141–163). New York: Raven Press.

[42] Ferber, R. E., & Kryger, M. H. (1995). Principles and practice of sleep medicine in the child. Philadelphia: Saunders.

[43] Forsyth, B. W. C., & Canny, P. F. (1991). Perceptions of vulnerability 3 1/2 years after problems of feeding and crying behaviour in early infancy. Pediatrics, 88, 757–763.

[44] Forsyth, W. C. (1989). Colic and the effect of changing formulas: a double-blind, multiple-crossover study. J. Pediatr., 115, 521–526.

[45] France, K. G. (1994). Handling parents' concerns regarding the behavioural treatment of infant sleep disturbance. Behaviour Change, 11 (2), 101–109.

[46] France, K. G. (1992). Behaviour characteristics and security in sleep disturbed infants treated with extinction. Journal of Pediatric Psychology, 17 (4), 467–475.

[47] France, K. G. (1996). Fact, act and tact: A three-stage approach to treating the sleep problems of infants and toddlers. Child and Adolescent Psychiatric Clinics of North America, 5 (3), 581–599.

[48] Frodi, A. (1985). When empathy fails: aversive infant crying and child abuse. In B. M. L. C. F. Z. Bourkydis (Ed.), Infant crying. New York: Plenum Press.

[49] Gaylor, E. E., Goodlin-Jones, B. L., Burnham, M. M., & Anders, T. F. (1998, 2–5 April). Maternal perception of night awakenings and infant self-soothing behavior during the first year of life. Paper presented at the International Conference of Infant Studies, Atlanta, USA.

[50] Glod, C. A., Teicher, M. H., Hartman, C. R., & Harakal, T. (1997). Increased nocturnal activity and impaired sleep maintenance in abused children. J Am Acad Child Adolesc Psychiatry, 36 (9), 1236−43.

[51] Greenspan, S., & Lourie, R. S. (1981). Developmental structuralist approach to the classification of adaptive and pathologic personality organisations: infancy and early childhood. American Journal of Psychiatry, 138, 725−735.

[52] Hagekull, B., & Dahl, M. (1987). Infants with and without feeding difficulties: maternal experiences. International Journal of Eating Disorders., 6 (1), 83−98.

[53] Halpern, L. F., Anders, T. F., Coll, C. G., & Hua, J. (1994). Infant temperament: is there a relation to sleep-wake states and maternal nighttime behavior? J. Infant Behavior and Development, 17, 255−263.

[54] Hanks, H., Hobbs, C., Seymour, D., & Stratton, P. (1988). Infants who fail to thrive: An intervention for poor feeding practises. Journal of Reproductive and Infant Psychology, 6, 101−111.

[55] Harris, G. (1988). Determinants of the Introduction of Solid Food. Journal of Reproductive and Infant Psychology., 6, 241−249.

[56] Harris, G. (1993). Feeding problems and their treatment. In I. St. James-Roberts, G. Harris, & D. Messer (Eds.), Infant crying, feeding and sleeping: Development, problems and treatments. London: Harvester Wheatsheaf.

[57] Harris, G. (1997). Development of taste perception and appetite regulation. In G. Bremner, A. Slater, & G. Butterworth (Eds.), Infant Development: Recent Advances (pp. 9−30). Hove: Psychology Press.

[58] Haynes, C. F., Cutler, C., Gray, J., & Kempe, R. S. (1984). Hospitalized cases of nonorganic failure to thrive: The scope of the problem and short-term lay health visitor intervention. Child Abuse and Neglect, 8, 229−242.

[59] Heptinstall, E., Puckering, C., Skuse, D., Start, K., Zur-Szpiro, S., & Dowdney, L. (1987). Nutrition and mealtime behaviour in families of growth retarded children. Human Nutrition: Applied Nutrition, 41, 390−402.

[60] Hill, D. J., & Hosking, C. S. (1995). The colic debate (letter). Pediatrics, 96, 165.

[61] Hubbard, F. O. A., & van Ijzendoorn, M. H. (1991). Maternal unresponsiveness and infant crying across the first 9 months: a naturalistic longitudinal study. Infant Behavior and Development, 14, 299−312.

[62] Hwang, C. P., & Danielsson, B. (1985). Dicyclomine hydrochloride in infantile colic. BMJ, 291, 1014−1015.

[63] Illingworth, R. S., & Lister, J. (1964). The critical or sensitive period, with special refernce to certain feeding problems in infants and children. The Journal of Pediatrics, 65 (6), 839−848.

[64] Iwaniec, D., Herbert, M., & McNeish, A. (1985). Social work with failure to thrive children and their families. Part 2: Behavioural social work intervention. British Journal of Social Work, 15, 375−389.

[65] Jenkins, S., Owen, C., Bax, M., & Hart, H. (1984). Continuities of common behaviour problems in preschool children. Journal of Child Psychology and Psychiatry, 25 (1), 75−89.

[66] Jones, D. P., & Verduyn, C. M. (1983). Behavioural management of sleep problems. Archives of Diseases in Childhood, 58, 442−444.

[67] Kahn, A., Mozin, M. J., Rebuttat, E., Sottiaux, M., & Muller, M. F. (1989). Milk intolerance in children with persistent sleeplessness: a prospective double-blind crossover evaluation. Pediatrics, 84 (4), 595−603.

[68] Kaplan, B. J., McNicol, J., Conte, R. A., & Noghadom, H. K. (1987). Sleep disturbance in preschool-aged hyperactive and nonhyperactive children. Pediatrics, 80, 839−844.

[69] Kedesky, J., & Budd, K. S. (1998). Childhood feeding disorders. Baltimore: Paul H Brookes Publishing Co.

[70] Keener, M. A., & Zeanah, C. H. A., T. F. (1988). Infant temperament, sleep organization, and nighttime parental intervention. Pediatrics, 81 (6), 762–771.

[71] Kessler, D. B., & Dawson, P. (1998). Failure to thrive and pediatric undernutrition. Baltimore: Paul H Brookes Publishing Co.

[72] Larson, K., & Ayllon, T. (1990). The effects of contingent music and differential reinforcement on infantile colic. Behav. Res. Ther., 28, 119–125.

[73] Lehtonen, L., Gormally, S., & Barr, R. G. (in press). Clinical pies, etiology and outcome in infants presenting with early increased crying. In R. G. Barr, B. Hopkins, & J. Green (Eds.), Crying as a signal, a sign and a symptom: Developmental and clinical aspects of early crying behavior: MacKeith Press. Lewis, M. (1992). Individual differences in response to stress. Pediatrics, 90 (3), 487–490.

[74] Lindberg, L. (1994). Early Feeding Problems: A developmental perspective. Uppsala: Acta Universitatis Upsaliensis; Comprehensive Summaries of Uppsala Dissertations from the Faculty of Social Sciences.

[75] Lindberg, L., Bohlin, G., & Hagekull, B. (1991). Early feeding problems in a normal population. International Journal of Eating Disorders, 10, 395–405.

[76] Lindberg, L., Bohlin, G., Hagekull, B., & Palmerus, K. (1996). Interactions between mothers and infants showing food refusal. Infant Mental Health Journal, 17, 334–347.

[77] Linscheid, T. R., & Rasnake, L. K. (1985). Behavioral approaches to the treatment of failure to thrive. In D. Drotar (Ed.), New directions in failure to thrive: implications for reasearch (pp. 279–294). New York: Plenum.

[78] Lothe, L., Lindberg, T., & Jakobsson, I. (1982). Cow's milk formula as a cause of infantile colic: a double-blind study. Pediatrics, 70 No.1, 7–10.

[79] Lozoff, B., & Zuckerman, B. (1988). Sleep problems in children. Pediatrics in review, 10 (1), 17–24.

[80] Lucassen, P. L. B. J., Assendelft, W. J. J., Gubbels, J. W., van Eijk, J. T. M., van Gelfrop, W. J., & Knuistingh Neven, A. (1998). Effectiveness of treatments for infantile colic: systematic review. British Medical Journal, 316, 1563–1569.

[81] Mathisen, B., Skuse, D., Wolke, D., & Reilly, S. (1989). Oral-motor dysfunction and growth retardation amongst inner-city infants. Developmental Medicine and Child Neurology, 31, 293–302.

[82] McDonough, S. C., Rosenblum, K., DeVoe, E., Gahagan, S., & Sameroff, A. (1998, 2–5 April). Parent concerns about infant regulatory problems: Excessive crying, sleep problems, and feeding difficulties. Paper presented at the International Conference of Infant Studies, Atlanta, USA.

[83] McMillen, I., Kok, J., Adamson, T., & Deayton, J. (1991). Development of circadian sleep wake rhythms in preterm and full term infants. Pediatric Research, 29 (4), 381–384.

[84] Messer, D., & Parker, C. (1998). Intants' sleep: Patterns and problems. In C. A. Niven & A. Walker (Eds.), Current issues in infancy and parenthood (Vol. 3, pp. 218–237). Oxford: Butterworth-Heinemann.

[85] Messer, D., & Richards, M. (1993). The development of sleeping difficulties. In I. St. James-Roberts, G. Harris, & D. Messer (Eds.), Infant crying, feeding and sleeping – development, problems and treatments . London: Harvester-Wheatsheaf.

[86] Messer, D. J., Lauder, L., & Humphrey, S. (1994). The effectiveness of group therapy in treating children's sleeping problems. Child: care, health and development, 20, 267–277.

[87] Miller, A. R., & Barr, R. G. (1991). Infantile colic. Is it a gut issue? Pediatric Clinics of North America, 38 (6), 1407–1423.

[88] Miller, A. R., Barr, R. G., & Eaton, W. O. (1993). Crying and motor behavior of six-week-old infants and postpartum maternal mood. Pediatrics, 92 No. 4, 551–558.

[89] Minde, K., Faucon, A., & Falkner, S. (1994). Sleep problems in toddlers: effects of treatment on their daytime behavior. J Am Acad Child Adolesc Psychiatry, 33 (8), 1114–21.

[90] Minde, K., Popiel, K., Leos, N., Falkner, S., Parker, K., & Handley-Derry, M. (1993). The evaluation and treatment of sleep disturbances in young children. Journal of Child Psychology and Psychiatry, 34, 521−533.

[91] Mindell, J. A. (1993). Sleep disorders in children. Health Psychology, 12 (2), 151−162.

[92] Mindell, J. A., & Durand, V. M. (1993). Treatment of childhood sleep disorders: Generalization across disorders and effects on family members. Special Issue: Interventions in pediatric psychology. Journal of Pediatric Psychology, 18(6), 731−750.

[93] Murray, L., Stanley, C., Hooper, R., King, F., & Fiori-Cowley, A. (1996). The role of infant factors in postnatal depression and mother-infant interactions. Developmental Medicine and Child Neurology, 38, 109−119.

[94] Owens, E. B., & Shaw, D. S. (1998, 2−5 April). Relations between infant irritability and maternal responsiveness in low-income families. Paper presented at the International Conference of Infant Studies, Atlanta, USA.

[95] Owens-Stively, J., Frank, N., Smith, A., Hagino, O., Spirito, A., Arrigan, M., & Alario, A. J. (1997). Child temperament, parenting discipline style, and daytime behavior in childhood sleep disorders [In Process Citation]. J Dev Behav Pediatr, 18 (5), 314−21.

[96] Papousek, M., & Papousek, H. (1996). Infant colic, state regulation, and interaction with parents: A systems approach. In M. H. Bornstein & J. L. Genevro (Eds.), Child development and behavioral pediatrics: Towards understanding children and health (pp. 11−33). Hillsdale: Lawrence Erlbaum Associates.

[97] American Association of Pediatrics. (1993). Shaken Baby Syndrome: inflicted cerebral trauma. Pediatrics, 92, 872−875.

[98] Pinilla, T., & Birch, L. L. (1993). Help me make it through the night: behavioral entrainment of breast-fed infants' sleep patterns. Pediatrics, 91, 436−444.

[99] Pollock, J. I. (1992). Predictors and long-term associations of reported sleeping difficulties in infancy. Journal of Reproductive and Infant Psychology, 10, 151−168.

[100] Zero to Three/National Center of Clinical Infant Programs. (1994). Diagnostic classification of mental health and developmental disorders of infancy and early childhood. Arlington: Author.

[101] Räihä, H., Lehtonen, L., Korhonen, T., & Korvenranta, H. (1996). Family life 1 year after infantile colic. Archives of Pediatrics and Adolescent Medicine, 150, 1032−1036.

[102] Ramsay, M. (1995). Feeding disorder and failure to thrive. Child and Adolescent Psychiatric Clinics of North America, 4 (3), 605−616.

[103] Reilly, S., Skuse, D., Mathisen, B., & Wolke, D. (1995). The objective rating of oral-motor functions during feeding. Dysphagia, 10, 177−191.

[104] Reilly, S. M., Skuse, D. H., Wolke, D., & Stevenson, J. (in press). Oral motor dysfunction in children who fail to thrive: Organic or non-organic? Developmental Medicine and Child Neurology.

[105] Richman, N. (1985b). A double blind drug trial of sleep problems in young children. Journal of Child Psychology and Psychiatry, 26, 591−598.

[106] Richman, N., Douglas, J., Hunt, H., Lansdown, R., & Levere, R. (1985). Behavioural methods in the treatment of sleep disorders − a pilot study. Journal of Child Psychology and Psychiatry, 26, 581−590.

[107] Rickert, V. I., & Johnson, M. (1988). Reducing nocturnal awakening and crying episodes in infants and young children: A comparison between scheduled awakenings and systematic ignoring. Pediatrics, 81, 203−212.

[108] Robert-Tissot, C., Cramer, B., Stern, D. N., Serpa, S. R., et al. (1996). Outcome evaluation in brief mother-infant psychotherapies: Report on 75 cases. Infant Mental Health Journal, 17 (2), 97−114.

[109] Robert-Tissot, C., & Cramer, B. (1998). When parents contribute to the choice of treatment. Infant Mental Health Journal, 19 (2), 245−259.

[110] Rydell, A.-M., Dahl, M., & Sundelin, C. (1995). Characteristics of school children who are choosy eaters. The Journal of Genetic Psychology, 156, 217−229.

[111] Sadeh, A. (1994). Assessment of Intervention for infant night waking: parental reports and activity-based home monitoring. Journal of Consulting and Clinical Psychology, 62 (1), 63−68.

[112] Sagi, A., Tirosh, E., Ziv, Y., Guttmann, S., & Lavie, P. (1998, 2−5 April). Attachment and sleep patterns in the first year of life. Paper presented at the International Conference of Infant Studies, Atlanta, USA.

[113] Sanger, S., Weir, K., & Churchill, R. (1981). Treatment of sleep problems: The use of behavioural modifications techniques by health visitors. Health Visitor, 54, 421−424.

[114] Sarimski, K. (1993). Aufrechterhaltung von Schlafstörungen im frühen Kindesalter: Entwicklungspsychopathologisches Modell und Pilot-Studie. Praxis für Kinderpsychologie und Kinderpsychiatrie, 42, 2−8.

[115] Satter, E. (1995). Feeding dynamics: Helping children to eat well. Journal of Pediatric Health, 9, 178−184.

[116] Scher, A., Epstein, R., Sadeh, A., Tirosh, E., & Lavie, P. (1992). Toddler's sleep and temperament: reporting bias or a valid link? a research note. Journal of Child Psychology and Psychiatry, 33 (7), 1249−1254.

[117] Seymour, F. W., Bayfield, G., Brock, P., & During, M. (1983). Management of night waking in young children. Australian Journal of Family Therapy, 4, 217−223.

[118] Seymour, F. W., Brock, P., During, M., & Poole, G. (1989). Reducing sleep disruptions in young children: evaluation of therapist-guided and written information approaches: a brief report. Journal of Child Psychology and Psychiatry, 30, 913−18.

[119] Shimada, M., Segawa, M., Higurashi, M., & Akamatsu, H. (1993). Development of the sleep and wakefulness rhythm in preterm infants discharged from a neonatal care unit. Pediatric Research, 33 (2), 159−163.

[120] Simonoff, E. A., & Stores, G. (1987). Controlled trial of trimeprazine tartrate for night waking. Archives of Disease in Childhood, 62, 253−257.

[121] Skuse, D. (1993). Epidemiologic and definitional issues in failure to thrive. Child and Adolescent Psychiatric Clinics of North America, 2 No. 1, 37−59.

[122] Skuse, D., Reilly, S., & Wolke, D. (1994a). Psychological adversity and growth during infancy. European Journal of Clinical Nutrition, 48, 113−130.

[123] Skuse, D., Pickles, A., Wolke, D., & Reilly, S. (1994b). Postnatal growth and mental development: evidence for a "sensitive period". Journal of Child Psychology and Psychiatry, 35, 521−545.

[124] Skuse, D., Stevenson, J., Reilly, S., & Mathisen, B. (1995). Schedule for oral-motor assessment (SOMA): Methods of validation. Dysphagia, 10, 192−202.

[125] Skuse, D., & Wolke, D. (1992). The nature and consequences of feeding problems in infants. In P. Cooper & A. Stein (Eds.), The nature and management of feeding problems and eating disorders in young people (pp. 1−25). New York: Harwood Academic Publishers.

[126] Skuse, D., Wolke, D., & Reilly, S. (1992). Failure to thrive. Clinical and developmental aspects. In H. Remschmidt & M. Schmidt (Eds.), Child and youth psychiatry. European perspectives. Vol. II: developmental psychopathology (pp. 46−71). Stuttgart: Hans Huber.

[127] St James-Roberts, I. (1992). Measuring infant crying and its social perception and impact. ACPP Review & Newsletter, 14 No. 3, 130−133.

[128] St. James-Roberts, I., & Halil, T. (1991). Infant crying patterns in the first year: normal community and clinical findings. Journal of Child Psychology and Psychiatry, 32 (6), 951−968.

[129] Stein, A., Woolley, H., Cooper, S. D., & Fairburn, C. G. (1994). An observational study of mothers with eating disorders and their infants. Journal of Child Psychology and Psychiatry, 35, 733−748.

[130] Stevenson, J. (1993). Sleep disturbance in children and its relationship to non-sleep behaviour problems. In I. St.James-Roberts, G. Harris, & D. Messer (Eds.), Infant crying, feeding and

sleeping: Development, problems and treatments (p 174−193). London: Harvester Wheat-sheaf.

[131] Stoleru, S., Nottelmann, E. D., Belmont, B., & Ronsaville, D. (1997). Sleep problems in children of affectively ill mothers. J Child Psychol Psychiatry, 38 (7), 831−41.

[132] Stores, G. (1996). Practitioner review: assessment and treatment of sleep disorders in children and adolescents. Journal of Child Psychology and Psychiatry, 37 (8), 907−925.

[133] Sullivan, P., & Rosenbloom, L. (Eds.). (1996). Feeding the disabled child. (Vol. 140). London: Clinics in Developmental Medicine.

[134] Thomas, J. M., & Clark, R. (1998). Disruptive behavior in the very young child: Diagnostic classification: 0−3 Guides classification of risk factors and relational interventions. Infant Mental Health Journal, 19 (2), 229−244.

[135] Tirosh, E., Scher, A., Sadeh, A., Jaffe, M., Rubin, A., & Lavie, P. (1993). The effects of illness on sleep behaviour in infants. Eur J Pediatr, 152 (1), 15−17.

[136] Trevathen, C. (1987). Sharing makes sense: intersubjectivity and the making of an infant's meaning. In R. Steele & T. Threadgold (Eds.), Language topics in Honor of Michael Halliday (Vol. 1, pp. 177−199). Philadelphia: John Benjamins.

[137] Tuchman, D. M., & Walter, R. S. (1994). Disorders of feeding and swallowing in infants and children: Pathophysiology, diagnosis and treatment. San Diego: Singular Publishing.

[138] Ungerer, J. A., Sigman, M., Beckwith, L., Cohen, S. E., & Parmelee, A. H. (1983). Sleep behavior of preterm children at three years of age. Developmental Medicine and Child Neurology, 25, 297−304.

[139] van den Boom, D. (1988). Neonatal irritability and the development of attachment: observation and intervention. Leiden: University of Leiden Ph.D. Dissertation.

[140] van der Maas, H. L. J., & Hopkins, B. (1998). Developmental transitions: what is new? British Journal of Developmental Psychology, 16, 1−14.

[141] van Izjendoorn, M., & Schuengel, C. (in press). The development of attachment relationships: infancy and beyond. In D. Messer & S. Millar (Eds.), Developmental Psychology. London: Arnold.

[142] von Hofacker, N., & Papousek, M. (1998). Disorders of excessive crying, feeding, and sleeping: The Munich Interdisciplinary Research and Intervention Program. Infant Mental Health Journal, 19 (2), 180−201.

[143] Weir, I. K., & Dinnick, S. (1988). Behaviour modification in the treatment of sleep problems occurring in young children: A controlled trail using health visitors as therapists. Child: Care, Health and Development, 14, 355−367.

[144] Weissbluth, M. (1987). Sleep and the colicky infant. In C. Guilleminault (Ed.), Sleep and its disorders in children. New York: Raven Press.

[145] Wessel, M. A., Cobb, J. C., Jackson, E. B., Harris, G. S., & Detwiler, A. C. (1954). Paroxysmal fussing in infancy, sometimes called "colic". Pediatrics, 14 No. 5, 421−434.

[146] Wilensky, D. S., Ginsberg, G., Altman, M., Tulchinsky, T. H., Yishay, F. B., & Auerbach, J. (1996). A community based study of failure to thrive in Israel. Archives of Disease in Childhood, 75, 145−148.

[147] Wolff, P. H. (1987). The development of behavioral states and the expression of emotions in early infancy. London: University of Chicago Press.

[148] Wolke, D. (1986a). The Feeding Interaction Scale (FIS)-Manual. From D. Wolke, University of Hertfordshire, Department of Psychology, College Lane, Hatfield, Herts, England.

[149] Wolke, D. (1986b). Play Observation Scheme and Emotion Rating (POSER)-Manual. From D. Wolke, University of Hertfordshire, Department of Psychology, College Lane, Hatfield, Herts, England.

[150] Wolke, D. (1987). Environmental neonatology (Annotation). Archives of Disease in Childhood, 62, 987−988.

[151] Wolke, D. (1990). Schwierige Säuglinge: Wirklichkeit oder Einbildung? In J. M. Pachler & H. M. Straßburg (Eds.), Der unruhige Säugling. Fortschritte der Sozialpädiatrie 13 (pp. 70−88). Lübeck: Hansisches Verlagskontor.

[152] Wolke, D. (1993). The treatment of problem crying behaviour. In I. St. James-Roberts, G. Harris, & D. Messer (Eds.), Infant Crying, Feeding and Sleeping: Development, Problems and Treatments (pp. 47−79). Hemel Hempstead: Harvester-Wheatsheaf.

[153] Wolke, D. (1994a). Feeding and sleeping across the lifespan. In M. Rutter & D. Hay (Eds.), Development through life: a handbook for clinicians (pp. 517−557). Oxford: Blackwell Scientific Publications.

[154] Wolke, D. (1995). Einschlaf- und Durchschlafprobleme bei biologischen Risikokindern und gesunden Vorschulkindern. In C. Becker-Carus (Ed.), Fortschritte der Schlafmedizin. Serie: Forum der Schlafmedizin (pp. 67−80). Münster-Hamburg: Lit-Verlag.

[155] Wolke, D. (1995a). Wo die klassische Pädiatrie an ihre Grenzen stößt: Die Erklärung und Behandlung von Regulationsstörungen bei Kindern. In K. Pawlik (Ed.), Bericht des 39. Kongreß der Deutschen Gesellschaft für Psychologie (pp. 469−476). Göttingen: Hogrefe.

[156] Wolke, D. (1996a). Probleme bei Neugeborenen und Kleinkindern. In J. Margraf (Ed.), Lehrbuch der Verhaltenstherapie (Vol. 2, pp. 363−380). Heidelberg: Springer.

[157] Wolke, D. (1996b). Failure to thrive: the myth of maternal deprivation syndrome. The Signal: Newsletter of the World Association for Infant Mental Health, 4, 1−6.

[158] Wolke, D. (1997). Die Entwicklung und Behandlung von Schlafproblemen und exzessivem Schreien im Vorschulalter. In F. Petermann (Ed.), Kinder-Verhaltenstherapie: Grundlagen und Anwendungen (pp. 154−203). Baltmannsweiler: Schneider-Verl. Hohengehren.

[159] Wolke, D. (1997b). Einschlafprobleme und -störungen durch Fehlen eines klaren Schafrituals (Chap. X-3.3). In H. Schulz (Ed.), Kompendium Schlafmedizin (der Deutschen Gesellschaft für Schlafforschung und Schlafmedizin. Landsberg a. Lech: ecomed Verlag.

[160] Wolke, D. (1997c). Kindliche Insomnie: Schlafstörungen aufgrund der Verstärkung von nächtlichem Aufwachen (Chap. X-3.4). In H. Schulz (Ed.), Kompendium Schlafmedizin (der Deutschen Gesellschaft für Schlafforschung und Schlafmedizin). Landsberg a. Lech: ecomed Verlag.

[161] Wolke, D. (1998a). Premature babies and the Special Care Baby Unit (SCBU)/Neonatal Intensive Care Unit (NICU): Environmental, medical and developmental considerations. In C. A. Niven & A. Walker (Eds.), Current issues in infancy and parenthood (Vol. 3, pp. 255−281). Oxford: Butterworth-Heinemann.

[162] Wolke, D. (1998b). Schlafstörungen bedingt durch nächtliches Essen und Trinken (Kap X-3.1). In H. Schulz (Ed.), Kompedium Schlafmedizin (Vol. 2. Reg. Lfg. 6/98,). Landsberg a. Lech: ecomed Verlag.

[163] Wolke, D., & Eldridge, T. (1998). The environment of care. In A. G. M. Campbell & N. McIntosh (Eds.), Forfar and Arneil's Textbook of Paediatrics (5 ed.). Edinburgh: Churchill Livingstone.

[164] Wolke, D., Gray, P., & Meyer, R. (1994b). Excessive infant crying: a controlled study of mothers helping mothers. Pediatrics, 94, 322−332.

[165] Wolke, D., & Messer, D. (submitted). Development of sleeping problems and their treatment in childhood. Journal of Psychosomatic Research.

[166] Wolke, D., & Meyer, R. (1995). The colic debate. Pediatrics, 96, 165−166.

[167] Wolke, D., & Meyer, R. (1998). Excessive infant crying and later behaviour problems: Findings of The Bavarian Longitudinal Study (BLS), Abstracts of papers presented at the Eleventh International Conference on Infant Studies Atlanta, Georgia, April 2−5, 1998. Infant Behavior and Development, 21 (Special ICIS Issue), 114.

[168] Wolke, D., & Skuse, D. (1992). The management of infant feeding problems. In P. J. Cooper & A. Stein (Eds.), Feeding problems and eating disorders in children and adolescents. Chur: Harwood Academic Publishers.

[169] Wolke, D., Meyer, R., & Gray, P. (1994d). Validity of the crying pattern questionnaire in a sample of excessively crying babies. J. of Reproductive and Infant Psychology, 12, 105–114.

[170] Wolke, D., Meyer, R., Ohrt, B., & Riegel, K. (1994a). Häufigkeit und Persistenz von Ein- und Durchschlafproblemen im Vorschulalter: Ergebnisse einer prospektiven Untersuchung an einer repräsentativen Stichprobe in Bayern. Praxis der Kinderpsychologie und Kinderpsychiatrie, 43, 331–339.

[171] Wolke, D., Meyer, R., Ohrt, B., & Riegel, K. (1994c). Prevalence and risk factors for infant excessive crying at 5 month of age. In W. Koops, B. Hopkins, & P. Engelen (Eds.), Abstract of the 13th Biennial Meeting of the International Society for the Study of Behavioural Development (pp. 152). Leiden (The Netherlands): Logon Publications.

[172] Wolke, D., Meyer, R., Ohrt, B., & Riegel, K. (1995). Co-Morbidity of crying and feeding problems with sleeping problems in infancy: Concurrent and predictive associations. Early Development and Parenting, 4, 191–207.

[173] Wolke, D., Meyer, R., Ohrt, B., & Riegel, K. (1995b). The incidence of sleeping problems in preterm and fullterm infants discharged from neonatal special care units: An epidemiological longitudinal study. Journal of Child Psychology and Psychiatry, 36, 203–223.

[174] Wolke, D., & Skuse, D. (1992). The management of infant feeding problems. In P. J. Cooper & A. Stein (Eds.), Feeding problems and eating disorders in children and adolescents (pp. 27–59). Chur: Harwood Academic Publishers.

[175] Wolke, D., Skuse, D., & Mathisen, B. (1990). Behavioral style in failure to thrive infants – a preliminary communication. Journal of Pediatric Psychology, 15, 237–254.

[176] Wolke, D., Soehne, B., Ohrt, B., Riegel, K., & Oesterlund, K. (1998). An epidemiological study of sleeping problems and feeding experience of preterm and fullterm children in South Finland: Comparison to a South German population sample. Journal of Pediatrics, 133.

[177] Wolke, D., & St. James-Roberts, I. (1987). Multi-method measurement of the early parent-infant system with easy and difficult newborns. In H. Rauh & H. C. Steinhausen (Eds.), Psychobiology and Early Development (pp. 49–70). Amsterdam: North-Holland/Elsevier.

[178] Wright, P. (1993). Mothers' ideas about feeding in early infancy. In I. St. James-Roberts, G. Harris, & D. Messer (Eds.), Infant crying, feeding and sleeping. Development, problems and treatment (pp. 99–117). Hemel Hempstead (UK): Harvester Wheatsheaf.

[179] Zeskind, P. S., & Shingler, E. A. (1991). Child abusers' perceptual responses to newborn infant cries varying in pitch. Infant Behavior and Development, 14, 335–347.

[180] Zuckerman, B., Bauchner, H., Parker, S., & Cabral, H. (1990). Maternal depressive symptoms during pregnancy, and newborn irritability. Developmental and Behavioral Pediatrics, 11 No. 4, 190–194.

[181] Zuckerman, B., Stevenson, J., & Bailey, V. (1987). Sleep problems in early childhood: Continuities, predictive factors, and behavioral correlates. Pediatrics, 80, 664–671.

3.13 Discussion

Dr. Bergmann:

Some children go to sleep only when you put them to bed with something they love, or give them a pacifier. But when they lose it, you have to get up at night and give it back! So what should we do; how do you call them – transitional things or something?

Prof. Wolke:

Yes, transition objects. Well, you have got dummies and you have transition objects: Dummies are again social-class dependent, you find them more frequently in the lower socio-economic groups than in the higher socio-economic groups. I think the important thing is that in the first few months there is not a recipe about whether they should have a dummy or not or should be fed. But at a later age what actually happens is that you can get into a pattern: then you not only give a dummy, but you give a bottle. And these infants are dependent on it all the time, and you can run into two problems. The one problem is they can't sleep without the bottle, they have never learned to fall asleep. So you're ninety percent there, if in the evenings you do not give the dummy or you do not give the bottle directly before sleep but you give it, give a feed when the infant is awake − that is for wake time − and then have a procedure to put them into bed, and you can talk to them, but do not rock them out any more. And secondly you have to make clear that you have got a bed-time when they're tired, because very often we hear, "It doesn't work, I put him down and he won't sleep". The reason is: the infant hasn't slept during the night, has been kept up in the morning, then you put them down for an afternoon nap from four to six and you expect them to sleep again at seven-thirty! There is one principle: the longest period of sleep follows the longest period of waking. And that is also related to colic-crying. So it is important that you have to look at the pattern; you shouldn't give any advice just on the basis of knowing if they have a dummy or not. You need to know the whole daily routine, when they sleep, at what time they sleep and so on, and that is why they keep diaries which we have developed for 7 days a week, and from there we can look exactly at the pattern and change that.

Prof. Hopkins:
One remark: In my own experience from a follow- up study we did, three infants died of sudden infant death. And all three of them had these three aspects you have talked about, this co-morbidity − the crying problem, the feeding problem, and the sleeping problem − according to the parents. And they stuck out in that respect from the rest of the sample. I just want to know have any comments on that, the association of this co-morbidity with something like cot-death.

Prof. Wolke:
About the association with cot-death: I mean you would have to have an inquiry because you will have to have a very very large population to find epidemiological statistical associations. But one of the things is: you find for example in pre-term infants more cot-deaths, they have more respiratory problems, but on the other hand what we have found is: pre-term infants (or) those who are failing to thrive start sleeping through the night early on, they do not necessarily have sleeping prob-lems, but they may cry and they may not eat very much. I do not know whether you looked at your infants whether they were not growing appropriately for their age, because that is a warning signal that has only recently been discovered showing they are undernourished and might have feeding problems. But regarding the cot-death rates, the biggest invention wasn't a high-tech one, but it was changing the

sleeping position of the baby to lying on the back. But because the parents do not usually come to the hospital when their baby has died, I have not seen many infants who had suffered sudden infant death. Also most studies were not large enough to establish representative results. Nevertheless, I see it as a real warning-sign, in particular in pre-term infants or infants who are not eating enough early-on and still sleep very well, I think it is more of a warning sign than excessive crying. Excessive crying can lead to abuse and shaking-baby-syndrome, you know, because you get so angry you throw them out, that is the one extreme − but the "very good baby" is actually a very worrisome baby for me, because it doesn't demand very much; and if that is paired with parents who find that great and do not wake them up at night or to feed them, you get in a cycle of low-appetite development, less eating, not growing properly, and in particular pre-term babies who're already down and often small for their age, that is a very detrimental combination.

Dr. Bergmann:
I think that some of the associations with breast-feeding are transitional. Because we were no good breast-feeders, and since breast-feeding is getting uneventful and we know more and more how to do it, then some of the problems are lost. Mothers are not over-tired, and [Prof. Wolke: Not depressed.] they sleep enough at night, and the children are quiet, and they do not cry − I think it was our fault − that we were not able to do it in the right way!

Prof. Wolke:
Yes. There are actually two things. The one thing is: we found, in Finland, that breast-feeding and distress early on was not related to more sleeping-problems at 20 months or 56 months of age, while in Germany it was. The reason for that is that in Finland nearly every-one breast-fed, while in Germany particular mothers breast-fed. And one of the issues around sleeping I couldn't talk about is also in the evening about letting go, of the mothers, that they feel like it is an important thing, in particular if you have been working, that when you come home that you can't let go. So one of our most successful interventions is to use fathers, to ask fathers to bring them to bed. But what you have to make clear is that the mother goes out of the house, she has to go to a friend because otherwise she comes and says: "you can't do it, you can't let him cry like this" or something like that. The only problem then, again, is for the fathers, after some weeks the mother won't come back. [laughter]

Prof. Bergmann (Chair):
Thank you very much.

4 Educating parents in the nutrition of their infants. Objectives and communication

Renate L. Bergmann, Karl E. Bergmann, Joachim W. Dudenhausen

One of the main goals in the nutritional education of parents in our modern world is to establish breast milk as the standard nutrition of all infants. A second objective of nutritional education is the weaning process and the introduction of suitable weaning foods.

The emergence of scientifically-based paediatric nutrition at the beginning of the last century displaced more behavioural and cultural approaches to nutrition. The benefits of breastfeeding in terms of infant morbidity and mortality were recognised. To promote and establish breastfeeding as a safe and easy nutritional method, new breastfeeding rules were propagated in Germany (Czerny, 1906, Manz, 1997) which required a baby to be put to breast according to a strict time schedule with the aim of forming an obedient personality from the first moment. Mothers and infants were separated after delivery. It was postulated that the first mother-infant contact should not occur before 24 hours after delivery, then the infant had to be attached alternatively to just one of both breasts every 4 hours with a night rest of 8 hours. These strict rules diminished breast-feeding prevalence until the 1970s.

Coincidental with this development, infant mortality declined rapidly, mainly because of improvements in artificial feeding, infant formulas, infant care and hygiene, and in the control of infectious diseases.

An important contribution to this development came from the Kaiserin Auguste Victoria-Haus (KAVH), which had been founded in 1909 as an Institute to "control for infant mortality in the German Reich". The mission of the Institute was to conduct research on infant nutrition, morbidity and mortality, while observing and studying pregnant women, newborns and infants (M Stürzbecher 1989).

First head of the KAVH-Institute was Arthur Keller, followed after two years by Leo Langstein. Fritz Rott became the manager of the "Organisationsamt" of this Institute, a department responsible for the transfer of the scientific results into actions of welfare for mother and child. Since at that time there were no official social departments responsible for the care of mother and child, for well baby stations or maternity wards, single mothers, or foster children, the Institute had an important role in the health education of the population regarding child care and hygiene (L Ballowitz 1991).

A wide variety of teaching materials were developed for this purpose, e. g. leaflets, of which some hundred thousands were distributed each year. But, as the authors state, "the written word will never have the radical force, urgently needed to reach the goal. i. e. to teach the people this important topic of public health care". Therefore, they write, "visual materials, models and practical advice" had to accompany the verbal mediation. A travelling museum of child hygiene was developed, which could reach a vast majority of the population. Exhibition walls, pictures, tables, photos, wax models and other images concerning the topic mother and child were transported in special suitcases and exhibited at many places. Films and magic lantern shows featured the development, care and nutrition of the infant and toddler.

One of the favourite teaching aids was the "Atlas of the Hygiene of the Infant and Toddler" published in 1918, with its loose posters (fig. 4. 1), used e. g. in baby care classes, education centres and elementary schools (L Langstein, F Rott 1918). Huge teaching baskets contained celluloid dolls, and articles for baby hygiene. Paper patterns for sewing, knitting and crocheting of clothes for mother and child were developed, periodicals were distributed and sold, also booklets and books on the nutrition of infants and children, on baby exercise, on physical activities for children, and on concentration exercises. In a party game called "Baby hop" correct answers concerning baby care were rewarded and wrong answers playfully punished. The teaching materials and the activities of the Institute and the Organisation Department were a real boon to the society.

A directive approach prevailed in the educational methods at the beginning of the last century. People were demanded to behave in a way that was considered beneficial for their own well-being and for the sake of the society. Maria Montessori was one of the first doctors and educators who emphasized the importance of the learning drive of the child for the learning process (B Broese 1970). Demand as the driving force for the gain in knowledge and competence is now accepted by modern pedagogy as well as by the economy. According to the results of our survey of a representative sample of German mothers and their partners after delivery, over 90% considered breast feeding and infant nutrition as one of the top subjects for anticipatory guidance in pregnancy (R Bergmann et al. 2000).

In this case, parents might be considered the consumers of knowledge and competence. But the infants are the actual consumer of the food offered. Nature therefore has provided them with an intrinsic knowledge of their nutritional needs (Bergmann, Bergmann 1986). The energy requirement for maintenance and growth will drive them to look for food. The food seeking clues can be recognized and learnt by a responsive mother. In the first hour after delivery the newborn will latch on to the breast and suck intensively. The stimulation of the nipple and the emptying of the

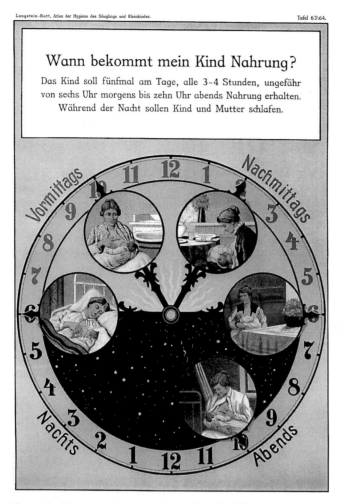

Fig. 4.1: Breast-feeding schedule. Langstein L, Rott F, 1918

breasts signal the infant's nutritional requirement to the maternal hormonal control centres and to local factors in the breasts (M Neville 2001).

Milk will be produced according to the demand of the infant and released by a let-down reflex, as soon as the infants latches on and the mother is relaxed and willing to breast feed. Beside nutritional needs, breast-feeding also satisfies the desire for non-nutritive suckling.

Demand feeding of the infant requires a close contact between both partners in this mother-child dyad. It requires rooming-in or even bedding-in, and an early start after delivery for a successful nursing (WHO 1996).

As a reaction to the disastrous spread of a bottle-feeding culture even in developing countries, at the world summit for children the World Health Organization and the United Children's Fund issued the Innocenty Declaration in Florence in 1990 on the protection, promotion and support of breast feeding in all member states (UNICEF/ WHO 1990). The Baby-Friendly-Hospital Initiative was launched in 1991 to promote breast-feeding as the standard nutrition in maternity facilities. The ten steps to successful breast feeding are based on scientific results and practical experience. They build the basis for the breast feeding education of mothers:

Step 1:

Have a written breast feeding policy, that is routinely communicated to all health care staff.

Step 2:

Train all health care staff in skills necessary to implement this policy.

Step 3:

Inform all pregnant women about the benefits and management of breast feeding.

Step 4:

Help mothers initiate breast feeding within half an hour after birth.

Step 5:

Show mothers how to breast feed and how to maintain lactation even when they are separated from their infants.

Step 6:

Give newborns no food or drink other than breast milk unless medically indicated.

Step 7:

Practice rooming in − allow mothers and infants to remain together 24 hours a day.

Step 8:

Encourage breast-feeding on demand.

Step 9:

Give no artificial teats or pacifiers to breast-feeding infants.

Step 10:

Foster the establishment of breast-feeding support groups and refer mothers to them on discharge from the hospital or clinic.

Simple cartoons were prepared for demonstrations, which could be easily copied and distributed, e. g. fig 4.2. The quality control requires 80% of mothers to know and to behave according to these rules. In Germany, health insurance companies pay for the home visits of midwifes who offer practical advice and help to the mother

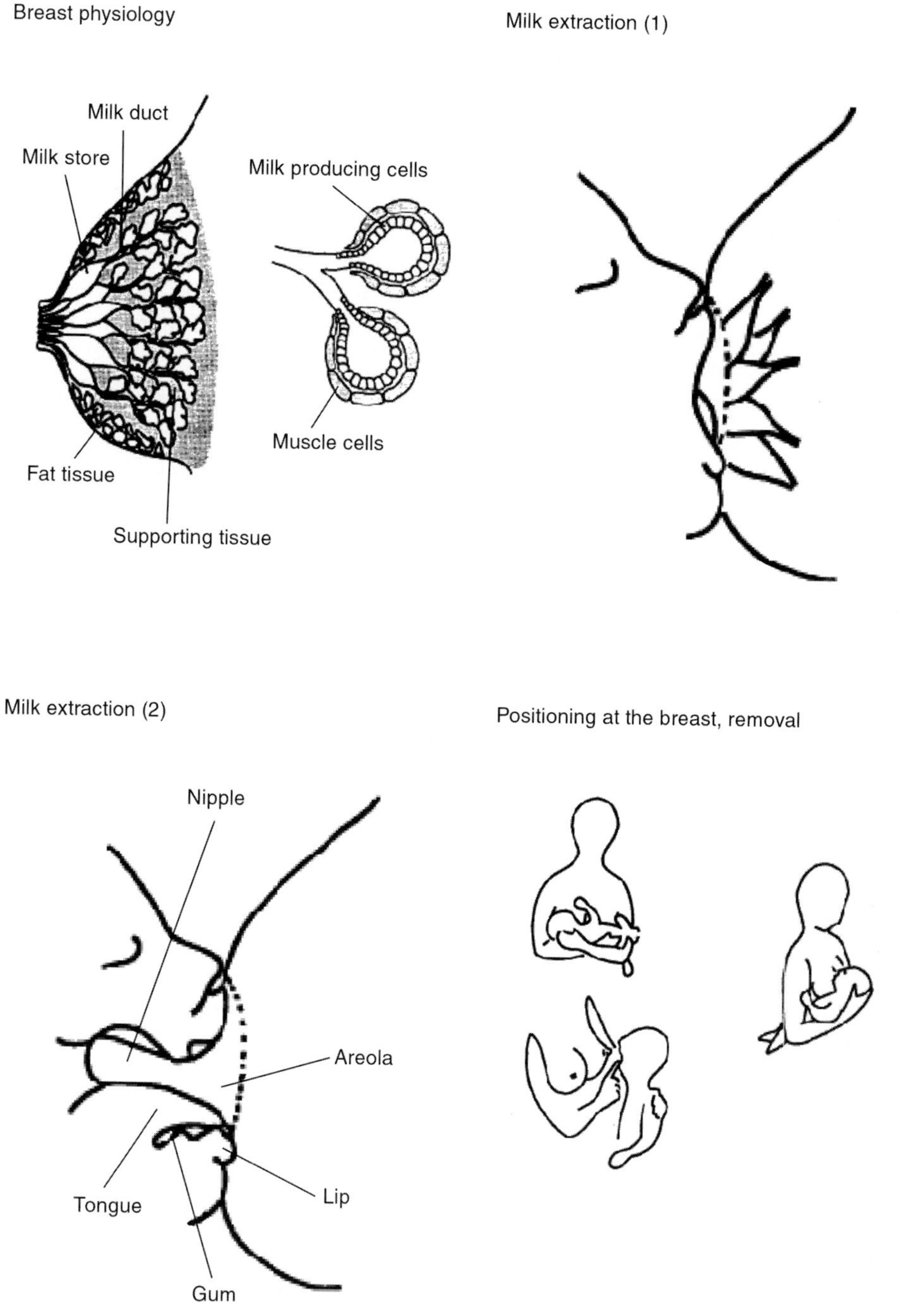

Breast physiology

Milk extraction (1)

Milk duct

Milk store

Milk producing cells

Muscle cells

Fat tissue

Supporting tissue

Milk extraction (2)

Positioning at the breast, removal

Nipple

Areola

Tongue

Lip

Gum

Fig. 4.2: Breast physiology, milk extraction, positioning and removal from the breast. Vinter TD, 1993

as long as they are breast feeding (WHO 1996). As the breast feeding culture is spreading again in our developed countries, expectant mothers can observe other mothers while they are feeding. Even children adapt this nursing behaviour as the standard and learn by playing the mothering game.

Parents have to learn that mother's milk – although it is considered to be the perfect food for infants – has to be supplemented with some vitamins and minerals to avoid marginal nutrition or nutritional deficiencies. Although not every infant might profit from these supplements, it is safer to give them to all infants rather than to screen for those who really need them, e. g. the vitamins K and D, and the trace elements fluoride and iron. Iodine is transferred to breast-milk, therefore breastfeeding mothers should take a supplement.

The next critical phase for nutritional education of parents is weaning – the introduction of solid food or *beikost*. Parents should offer this new experience as soon as the infant is developmentally ready to take food from a spoon by the lips, to push mashed food with the tongue and anterior hard palate, i. e. between 4–7 months (Stevenson 1979, Ayano 2000, Tamiura 2000). Some infants are curious and show a demand for new foods, but usually, the parents offer the new type of food first, and try to convince their infant of the new feeding technique, and to train it. The new taste experience is another problem. Infants have a sweet tooth and like sweet food. But in Germany, vegetables, especially mashed carrots, are traditionally the first solids introduced to the infant, potatoes and minced meat (for protein and iron) added to the menu after one and two weeks, respectively. Not all infants agree to it, because for some carrots taste bitter. Since the second recommended solids, introduced four weeks after the first menu, are sweet cereal paps with milk and fruit, some parents prefer to give this to reluctant infants first, and then the vegetable menu.

These first solids are usually finely mashed, later lumpy solids will be offered. When lumpy solids were not introduced until after 10 months of age, children were more difficult to feed and had more definite likes and dislikes later (Northstone 2001). This demonstrates that after the breast-feeding phase, the nutritional demands of the infant (hunger or thirst) are not the main driving forces for food intake. The pleasure of eating develops, which includes all kinds of satisfactions of their wants. Parents offer food and interact with the infant according to their knowledge and parental skills.

With the development of motor abilities, social skills and personality, there will be a progression in the eating development of the infant which parents can assist. Parents should therefore be educated in infant nutrition and in infant development. They should learn about things to look out for in development, they should learn how to deal with normal exploratory behaviour, with normal poor appetite, and how to overcome the tantrums of a toddler (Schmitt 1997). Their assuredness and responsiveness will then help them to establish good feeding behaviour, and to avoid habits that are hard to break, e. g. the permanent suckling from tea-bottles or the permanent nibbling of biscuits.

Who should teach parents these skills? In traditional large families this was the task of grandparents and other relatives. Our survey of parents after delivery showed that parents were not satisfied with this advice (Bergmann 2000). Times are changing, many of the old habits are out of date. Parents are eager to get advice for their child's development in advance ("anticipatory guidance"). They prefer to be taught by medical personnel. We therefore consider seminars in small groups of parents with infants of the same age to be best. Visual materials, videos, movies and models like those of the former KAVH can be used for demonstrations.

References

[1] Ayano R, Tamura F, Ohtsuka Y, Mukai Y: The development of normal feeding and swallowing: Showa Univerity study of feeding function. Int J Orofacial Myology 2000; 26: 24–32.

[2] Bergmann RL, Kamtsiuris P, Bergmann KE, Huber M, Dudenhausen JW: Kompetente Elternschaft: Erwartung von jungen Eltern an die Beratung in der Schwangerschaft und an die Entbindung. Z Geburtsh Neonatol 2000; 204: 60–67.

[3] Bergmann RL, Bergmann KE: Nutrition and growth in infancy. In F Falkner, JM Tanner: Human Growth. 2nd ed. Volume 3, Plenum Press New York, 1986:389–413.

[4] Broese B: Maria Montessori: eine kritische Würdigung ihrer Wirksamkeit anlässlich der 100. Wiederkehr ihres Geburtstages (Maria Montessori- a critical estimation of her effectiveness on the occasion of the 100th anniversary of her birth). Zschr ärztl Fortbild 1970; 64: 1175–1180.

[5] Czerny A, Keller A: Des Kindes Ernährung, Ernährungsstörungen und Ernährungstherapie: ein Handbuch für Ärzte. Vol 1. Deuticke, Leipzig, Vienna. 1906.

[6] Engle PL, Bentley M, Pelto G: The role of care in nutrition programmes: current research and a research agenda. Proc Nutr Soc 2000; 59: 25–35.

[7] Langstein L und Rott F: Atlas und Beiheft der Hygiene des Säuglings und Kleinkindes. Julius Springer 1918 Berlin. Reprint 1989, Schmidt-Römhild Lübeck.

[8] Ballowitz L: Leo Langstein. Biographische Daten und beruflicher Werdegang. In: Leonore Ballowitz (Ed.): Schriftenreihe zur Geschichte der Kinderheilkunde aus dem Archiv des Kaiserin Auguste Victoria Hauses (KAVH)- Berlin. Heft 8. Druck Humana Milchwerke Westfalen 1989, 42–50.

[9] Manz F, Manz I, Lennert T: Zur Geschichte der ärztlichen Stillempfehlungen in Deutschland. Monatsschr Kinderheilkd 1997; 145: 572–587.

[10] Neville MC: Anatomy and Physiology of Lactation. In RJ Schanler (ed) The Pediatric Clinics of North America. Breastfeeding 2001; I Part; The Evidence for Breastfeeding: 13–34.

[11] Northstone K, Emmett P, Nethersole F: The effect of age of introduction to lumpy solids on foods eaten and reported feeding difficulties at 6 and 15 months. J Human Nutr Diet 2001; 14: 43–54.

[12] Schmitt BD: Seven deadly sins of childhood: advising parents about difficult developmental phases. Child Abuse and Neglect 1987; 11: 421–432.

[13] Stevenson RD, Alleire JH: The development of normal feeding and swallowing. Pediatric Clinics of North America 1991; 38: 1439–1453.

[14] Stürzbecher M: Arthur Keller. Der erste ärztliche Direktor des Kaiserin Auguste Victoria Hauses. In: Leonore Ballowitz (Ed.): Schriftenreihe zur Geschichte der Kinderheilkunde aus

dem Archiv des Kaiserin Auguste Victoria Hauses (KAVH)- Berlin. Heft 6. Druck Humana Milchwerke Westfalen 1989, 42–50.

[15] Tamura F, Chigira A, Ishii H, Nishikata H, Mukai Y: Assessment of the development of hand and mouth coordination when taking food into the oral cavity. Int J Orofacial Myology 2000; 26: 33–43.

[16] Vinter TD: Breastfeeding. How to support success. WHO Copenhagen 1993.

[17] World Health Organisation: Promoting breastfeeding in health facilities. WHO Geneva and Wellstart International San Diego 1996.

5 Vaccinations

Sabine Reiter, Gernot Rasch, Christiane Meyer, Sieghart Dittmann,
Karl E. Bergmann

5.1 Introduction

5.1.1 The importance of vaccinations

The health and the life expectancy of children and their parents improved in the 20th century to an unprecedented degree. Levels of infant mortality in 2000 were one fiftieth of those in 1900, and child mortality is lower by a factor of 65. In 1900 the mortality of women aged between 20 and 45 years of age was above 25%, the mortality of men of this age was considerably higher, not least due to the effects of war, so that many children grew up without their own mother and father, often enough in orphanages. Today there are virtually no orphanages in Germany any more.

A significant contribution to the decline in mortality has been made by the work against infections. In addition to hygienic measures and effective medication, a crucial element of this success has been vaccinations both against infections that threaten individuals, and against epidemics which threaten the population as a whole. For example, in 1900 65 000 children died in Germany from whooping cough, diphtheria and rubella in one year (with a total population of 58 million). The influenza pandemic of 1918/19 led to 20 million deaths world-wide. During the last major polio epidemic in Germany, some 5000 people were infected. The dramatic rise in diphtheria in the former USSR and the polio epidemic of 1992 in the Netherlands and of 1996/97 in Albania demonstrate quite clearly that without the protection of vaccinations illnesses can return which were believed to have been vanquished long ago.

With the introduction of effective vaccinations it became possible both to provide individual protection against illness and also to provide population immunity in an epidemiological sense. The eradication of smallpox, the imminent elimination of poliomyelitis, which is expected to be confirmed in 2003, and the plans to eliminate measles by 2010 are examples of the strategic role of vaccinations in overcoming dangerous illness.

Taking vaccinations as an example it is possible to explain the important elements of an effective prevention strategy.

5.1.2 Obligatory vaccination

When smallpox vaccinations were introduced, the health policy makers were convinced that it was only possible to protect individuals, and above all the population as a whole by compulsory vaccinations. This strategy proved to be successful. In the then East Germany all other vaccinations were also made compulsory, so that after the eradication of smallpox in 1980 the large majority of the population were also sufficiently immunised against other infections.

5.1.3 Vaccinations as a voluntary contribution to prevention

With the eradication of smallpox, vaccinations against it were no longer required. But this had an undesirable knock-on effect, at least in Western Europe. For all other vaccinations and those subsequently introduced, strategies had to be devised to achieve high rates of vaccination. Since most of the vaccinations were initially provided by the public health service, it was possible to send official invitations out to individuals and families to attend. But for some years now the vaccinations have been carried out by family doctors, who cannot do this, and who are also legally obliged to explain all the possible negative effects involved. On top of this, the fee paid for the vaccinations is not satisfactory. In West Germany the rates of vaccination against many infectious diseases remained unsatisfactory. After the fall of the Berlin Wall and German unification vaccinations also became voluntary in east Germany.

5.1.4 Deficit analysis

In such a situation a deficit analysis is appropriate. This shows that in Germany the acceptability of vaccinations plays an important role. It is estimated that less than 2% of the population in Germany are strict opponents of vaccination. About 10% of parents are thought to be sceptical, that is they rejected individual vaccinations for their children. The majority of the general public are uninformed and thus feel insecure, or are unworried to simply blasé. Investigations of the causes for inadequate rates of vaccination show the following problems:

- Insufficient awareness of the dangers of infectious diseases.
- The knowledge of the benefits and the necessity of vaccinations is not only inadequate among the lay public, but also among many doctors.
- Vaccinations, and in particular boosters are often forgotten.
- Many parents are made to feel insecure by vaccination opponents. In particular midwives often advise against vaccinations.
- Parents are often worried about side-effects.
- Incorrect contraindications, such as a trivial infection, lead to important vaccinations being postponed and often enough then completely forgotten.

- In addition, the data situation regarding side-effects after vaccinations is unsatisfactory.
- Frequently vaccination damage is recognised by official bodies although this is not the case.
- The health insurance organisations do not all deal with the costs in the same way.
- Doctors often feel insecure about the problems of legal liability and are afraid that they run the risk of being sued for damages if they give vaccinations.
- Doctors can only charge very low fees for giving vaccinations.
- On the whole, preventive medicine has a very low standing in Germany.
- Vaccinations are not discussed enough, in particular not in schools.
- There are also problems arising from the state of the infrastructure, for example the poor availability of data about vaccination status.
- The various agencies active in preventive vaccination do not cooperate together well.
- Among practising physicians the lack of information is in part considerable.
- Social factors have an influence on participation in vaccination programmes, particularly social status, income, level of education, ethnicity, and family status (e. g. single parent, number of children, sibling ranking, age of parents).
- The family doctors have a big influence on vaccination participation: 85% of respondents would follow their advice.
- Doctor-patient contacts are not used frequently enough to check vaccination status and to provide booster vaccinations.

On the basis of these points, a 10-point programme was drawn up to increase acceptance of vaccinations.

5.2.10 Point Programme to Increase the Acceptance of Vaccinations and to Increase Rates of Vaccination in Germany-Preambel

Objectives and benefits of vaccinations

Vaccinations are the most important and most effective of medical preventive measures. Modern vaccinations are very compatible, and grave undesirable side-effects are only observed in very rare cases. The direct objective of vaccinations for individuals is to strengthen the natural immune system against invasive agents and to prevent an illness. Vaccinations protect against:

- Severe infectious illnesses which cannot the treated causally,
- Possible severe complications due to infectious illnesses,
- Complications due to severe basic illnesses,
- Infectious illnesses that can lead to severe damage to the unborn baby during pregnancy.

Achieving high rates of vaccination in the population mean that it is possible to break through the chain of infection and eliminate individual causes of illness at first regionally and finally world-wide. Vaccinations have very good cost-benefit effects and thus contribute to cutting costs in the health service.

The necessity for vaccinations
In view of the epidemiological situation – the world-wide re-emergence of infectious illnesses that had long been thought to have been eliminated, the increase in mobility, tourism and migration with the associated danger of transporting infectious illnesses from one region to another, combined with an unsatisfactory level of vaccination protection in Germany – mean that appropriate vaccination protection is about the most important preventive measure against numerous infectious illnesses. In international comparison, Germany has a rate of vaccination typical for a developing country. International health policy targets such as the eradication of poliomyelitis and the elimination of measles can only be achieved in Germany if the vaccination situation improves considerably.

The German structures involve subsidiarity and federalism. The various organisations and institutions therefore frequently do not concentrate on the population of Germany as a whole, but closely follow a remit to concentrate on individual protection or the collective protection of a specific region. Strategies for an intervention programme cannot be monolithic, but must combine the various viewpoints and fields of operation in a synergetic fashion.

This is not a matter of either individual or collective protection. Rather, vaccination programmes are a priority Public Health measure and offer effective individual prevention, and they must be implemented equally by all those with responsibility for protecting the health of the population, independent of regional and institutional allegiances.

1. **Concerted action "Vaccination": Concentrate and harmonise measures and activities at national and regional levels:**

- Establishment of a national vaccination programme to eliminate infectious illnesses, e. g. measles.
- A national consensus about the need for the vaccinations among all those involved in the health system (doctors, health insurances, legislature) to be established by a more intensive campaign of information and explanation.
- All relevant institutions at national and regional levels must participate actively with binding undertakings.
- Vaccination programmes are to be established which make efficient use of the available resources under the starting conditions.
- Existing networks must be expanded, made more efficient, and at the same time more transparent.
- The form and content of information and actions must be harmonised, because only then will they be effective and benefit from the brand recognition.

- It may be necessary to establish appropriate priorities in order to eliminate measles.

In Germany there are a number of institutions and organisations that are working successfully in preventive vaccination. But more effective cooperation, and the concentration of planned measures and harmonisation of preventive messages could, however, considerably improve the vaccination situation.

2. The epidemiological data situation is being improved by:

- The new law on protection against infections (IfSG) which came into effect on 1 Jan 2001, and which provides for improved compulsory registration of infectious diseases and vaccinations.
- An improved data situation for regional and age-related vaccination rates, antibody prevalences and morbidity rates for illnesses which can be prevented by vaccination.
- The integration of the topic of vaccination in existing sentinels and surveys.
- Setting up sentinels to register e. g. measles and travel-related diseases.
- Improved registration of vaccine side-effects.
- A nation-wide survey of the vaccination status of pre-school and school children by the public health service.
- A standardisation of the data recorded in screening tests by the public health service.

Reliable and detailed data help to increase the acceptance of vaccinations and enable rational discussion, as well as being necessary for the planning, implementation and evaluation of vaccination programmes, the policy consultancy and information campaigns both for the general public and physicians.

3. Removing infrastructure constraints:

- The STIKO recommendations should be implemented uniformly by all German Laender.
- The situation about the problems of liability for doctors giving vaccinations should be clarified so as to create security before the law.
- The public health service must be strengthened since it is the only organisation that can have a clear overview of the vaccination situation at the level of local authorities and at the same time has access to the sectors of the population who do not make use of the out-patient services.
- The cooperation between family doctors and the public health service must be improved.
- The vaccination status of the patients should be established by means of computer systems or smart cards, data should be collated.

Infrastructure constraints lead to insecurity in the general public and among doctors, and hinder an effective participation in vaccination programmes.

4. Creating incentives, improving the regulations about the costs of vaccinations and the organisation of the emoluments system:

- Standard acceptance of costs by all health insurance organisations.
- Costs for all vaccinations recommended by STIKO for Germany should not be a matter for discretionary decisions by the health insurers – they should be obliged to accept them.
- Reduction of vaccine costs by ordering economical large packs with standard suppliers for all types of health insurance system.
- Reduction of vaccine costs by changes to value-added tax rates (as in other European countries).
- Higher fees for giving vaccinations and for giving advice.
- Simple, standard charging procedures.
- Separate charging codes for each vaccination.
- Exclusion of vaccinations from budgeting systems.
- Bonus systems for doctors and patients.
- Payment by health insurers of costs for public health service vaccinations in problematic social areas and for special target groups.

The differing regulations about acceptance of costs of vaccines by the health insurance organisations and the varying organisation of the payment of doctor's fees are a constraint on increasing the rates of vaccination.

5. Improving medical training and in-job training:

- A vaccination course should be obligatory for all medical students, so that all future physicians are qualified in this field. This demand of the *Deutsche Ärztetag* of the past years should be implemented.
- Implementation of the motion passed at the *Bundesärztekammer* on 22. 08. 1997: Every physician should be able to carry out vaccinations of assured quality.
- General practitioners and internal specialists should be encouraged by professional organisations and health insurance bodies to provide vaccinations, in order to close the major gaps in coverage of the adult population.
- Quality assurance can be achieved by certifications and further training.
- Medical advice on travelling abroad must be standardised and quality controlled.
- More emphasis must be placed on the WHO Measles Elimination Programme at conferences and further training meetings.
- Vaccination further training events to be carried out by specialist associations, and professional bodies and organisations.

Family doctors and practising physicians have a key role to play in advising on and providing vaccinations. Their motivation and qualification are therefore the core elements of a successful preventive vaccination programme.

6. Vaccination advice and vaccination in accordance with STIKO recommendations as core of an active doctor-patient relationship:

- Use every contact between doctor and patient and all screening check-ups to check on vaccination protection and to carry out recommended vaccinations and boosters.
- Actively question patients about vaccination protection, if appropriate in the framework of marketing strategies.
- Under-7 and Year 1 check-ups should only be marked as completed when vaccination counselling has been included.
- Introduction of professional regulations under which patient can be actively invited and encouraged to return for booster vaccinations.
- (Re-)activation of vaccination counselling and vaccinations for Kindergarten entrants.
- Use of appropriate occasions (trips abroad, start of school, changing seasons) for vaccination counselling and vaccinations by the family doctor.
- Filling up gaps in the vaccination coverage through the public health service, in particular for patient groups that are not reached by the practising physicians.

Active marketing and the use of doctor-patient contacts to check up on vaccination status can increase patient awareness and thus increase the rates of vaccination.

7. Activating company and trade medical services to close the vaccination gap for adults:

- Motivation and qualification of doctors working in company and trade medical services for vaccinations.
- Use of doctor-patient contacts in the course of consultations in company and trade medical services for counselling on vaccinations, and giving booster jabs.
- Educational and information campaigns by the company and trade medical services.
- Systematic integration of vaccination information in company health education campaigns.

Company and trade doctors can easily contact healthy personnel. They can play an important role in providing information about vaccinations in companies, checking vaccination status and carrying out vaccinations.

8. Promoting vaccinations among prominently placed individuals outside the medical profession:

- Increased motivation and qualification of midwives, homecare and clinic staff, teachers, social workers, etc.
- Including the training and educational sectors in organised campaigns.

- Inclusion of non-medical role-models in information campaigns (finding out vaccination status, encouraging people to find out more about vaccinations and to take part in campaigns).
- Development of satisfactory information material for these campaigns.
- Inclusion of preventive vaccination as a topic in classes, including contributions by the public health service.

Lay people in the health and educational services can have a multiplication function, exercising considerable influence on children, young people and individual target groups. It is important that they are motivated to take part in vaccination campaigns and programmes.

9. **Motivation of the general public by means of personal communications, mass communications and action days:**

- Development of an effective coordination of personal communication, mass communication and action days.
- Identification of specific target groups and the development of appropriate programmes with clear, consistent messages.
- Promotion of the benefits for individuals and society of vaccinations, with information about the possible severe complications that can arise with illnesses that could be prevented by receiving vaccinations.
- Active approach to potential fears by means of increased information about the safety of vaccines.
- Active rebuttal of the false arguments of opponents of vaccinations.
- Organisation of action days, annual vaccination days, and pilot projects in combination with other information policies.

A variety of communication strategies and materials are needed to generate appropriate awareness in the general public, in accordance with the individual needs and interests of the various target groups.

10. **Agenda-setting in the media by:**

- Intensification of the contacts with journalists, in particular from television and radio.
- The preparation of suitable information material for the media.
- The systematic involvement of media representatives in preparing and implementing vaccination actions.
- Availability of increased information via the Internet.
- Propagating the vaccination message as part of Infotainment strategies.

If a topic is to attract broad attention, the in our modern information societies the media play a key role.

As a result of these measures the vaccination rates in Germany have increased considerably.

6 Healthy from the beginning: Promoting the mental and physical development, and preventing injuries of young children

A programme of the AOK Health Insurance Association to promote health in young and expectant families – Concept for one of several slide presentations for young parents

Karl E. Bergmann, Renate L. Bergmann, Sibylle Becker

Dear Parents,

If your child is now six months old, then the past 2 or 3 months were probably very special. Your child was in a good mood most of the time, had settled down into a daily rhythm, was happy to see you, and responded to your attention with boundless love.

But at this age things are gradually changing. Your child will soon be turning round and stretching out for objects which had been out of reach before, and will become more and more mobile. These are the first steps on the road towards independence, which after many years will see your child as a fully responsible adult. Accompanying this development is a considerable challenge for you. Because your child cannot yet understand the world, there are dangers on all sides. In the coming years there will be the risks of accidental injuries, and then later the various temptations that threaten to lure young people away their chosen path in life. You are now called on to rise to the challenge. For your child you are the highest authority, and the role model for what they will aspire to be.

Slides 6.1–6.2

Accidents pose a very great threat for small children. Most of them occur at home. They are often the result of the increasing independence and mobility of the children in an environment that is not yet familiar to them, coupled with irrepressible curiosity. Prevention consists of two components: providing a safe environment, and developing the competence of the parents and of the children.

Slide 6.3

Accidents are thus a wonderful example for parents to show how they can develop their parenting skills.

Slide 6.4

A leading German educationalist wrote that "Bringing up children is love and example and nothing else". On closer inspection, upbringing transmits love, bonding, knowledge, understanding of the world, of other people and of oneself, but also skills, culture, empathy, the ability to converse with other people, to live and work with them. Upbringing establishes relationships in the family and the living space of the child. It provides support for the child and sets boundaries. Most of these aspects play an important role when it comes to avoiding and preventing accidents.

Slide 6.5

When a child first begins to learn about its environment, then there are big dangers lurking everywhere. Even a completely normal setting for adults can be very risky for a child, simply because it does not know what the dangers are. The child can fall onto something, pick up an everyday object the wrong way or use it incorrectly, can get burnt or scalded, injured in road traffic, poisoned with pharmaceutical products, cleaning agents or cigarettes, can inhale small objects, or drown in shallow water.

Slides 6.6–6.11 optional
Slide 6.12

The level of development of personality plays an important role: Small children are very inquisitive and active. They are always on the move, and want to find out what they can about the little world around them. They are completely naive and know no dangers, they are clumsy and have a poor sense of balance. Their memory is short. They see themselves as the centre of the world.

Slide 6.13

A particular problem is that they are constantly learning to do new things, often to the surprise of their parents: They recognise distant objects and want to find out about them. They begin by turning to them, but are soon rolling, crawling, pulling themselves up into a standing position, they learn to stand without support, and then soon they can walk.

Slide 6.14

At this age the children move around faster and faster, and can act so quickly and unexpectedly that you can hardly take your eyes off your child for a second. Only a few weeks after taking their first steps they are getting everywhere. They can climb onto chairs, tables, sofas, and window sills, and are no longer content just to touch things they have seen. They have soon learnt to open containers, pull out drawers, turns knobs, switch switches, and to turn a key in a lock, take it out and then throw it in a waste-paper basket.

Slide 6.15

If a child is under careful supervision, then it is usually possible to avoid serious injuries. But you must be aware that this environment also harbours risks. The parents are often tired and exhausted, they may be concentrating on each other, perhaps having an argument, sometimes they will bring the pressures of work back home with them. Unexpected events such as separations, illness or even the death of people near them can make parents think of other things, to the detriment of their child. Visits or long trips can also give rise to risks. And when they have finally found a babysitter, so that they can have free hours together, it takes time before the babysitter is familiar with the risks of the home and the abilities of the child, so that here too there are risks of accidents.

Slide 6.16—6.23 optional

As soon as your child begins to crawl you would be well advised to look over the main accidents risks in your domestic environment. We have drawn up a checklist to help you make things secure for your child. The goal in particular is to avoid the serious or even life-threatening injuries. Bumps and bruises, on the other hand, may even be something your child can learn from. It is necessary to keep a sense of proportion. And even if a home has been made safe, it does not free you from the obligation of keeping a loving and watchful eye on your child.

Avoiding accidents would, of course, be much easier in a family with enough money to pay for everything it needed. But young families are rarely in such a fortunate financial situation. That often only comes much later on, when the children have left home and are standing on their own feet. And to be truthful, it is actually much nicer if things require some improvisation and are not so perfect to begin with.

Slide 6.24—6.25

Some people will find it easier in their well-ordered home and with an easy daily schedule to keep a good eye on their little bundle of energy. Even if few other people have to deal with your child and only a few people pay regular visits, it is easier for you to be parents and to care for the safety of your child. If it is possible, we would recommend avoiding hectic travels and to keep as much time as possible free for your child. If you are well organised you yourselves can create the preconditions that help to protect against accidents.

Slide 6.26

Your child should not become just a sideshow in your life, whatever the occupational demands. Make yourself familiar with the developments children go through. It might help to read a few chapters in a book or to buy a few of the magazines produced for young parents. If you identify any safety problems, do something about it right away.

Slide 6.27

Put some effort into ensuring an optimistic, friendly climate in the family. Support each other and help your child to learn. Always bear in mind that you are the most important people in the life of your child, and do your best to do justice to your obligations as parents.

Slide 6.28

Even after half a year, children can already learn a lot, but they generally have a very short memory: if you take something away from a 6-month-old baby, it will soon have forgotten that the object exists and simply play with something else. Three or four months later the situation is very different. At this age, children start to remember objects. Even if they cannot see them at that moment, they still know that the object exists. This enhanced memory improves their ability to learn and thus also your chance as parent to start helping the child to learn things. Rest assured that your child is completely good-natured, even though it wants to try out everything it can. Your child will react positively when it is praised for doing things the way that you like. You can use this to guide the behaviour of your child. It is fortunate that children at the end of their first year begin to develop fear of strange things and unfamiliar faces. This helps to protect them somewhat against the effects of rash actions – although it doesn't protect them completely. When they do bump themselves or fall over then they have the advantage that they are still very light, are well-cushioned, and have fairly elastic bones. Minor injuries usually heal well.

Slide 6.29

As their senses become more acute, and their mobility and agility improves, children also understand more of what is said to them and they are able to gain experience, which improves their safety in their normal environment.

Slide 6.30

As a rule, children naturally want to learn. They observe things more and more closely and gather experience by actively confronting everything in their surroundings, ...

Slide 6.31

... imitating things they have seen other people doing and watching how their parents react, and finally exercising their muscles by pulling themselves up, and climbing over things.

Slide 6.32

Encourage this development by offering your child opportunities to gain experience in its surroundings. The best way to do this is to develop a loving, trusting relationship with your child, in which you can talk, sing songs, and dance, also providing enough things to play with. Encourage the independence of your child and encourage its natural need to learn.

Slides 6.33, 6.34 optional,
Slide 6.35

One of the most interesting things for children to play with are their mom and dad. This offers something to climb on, to jump on, and to push and pull. Toys can be bought, but they can also be home-made. Children will happily play with egg boxes (perhaps they should be heated at 100 degrees in the oven beforehand and then allowed to cool), the cardboard centre of kitchen rolls, or empty plastic bottles.

Slides 6.36, 6.37 optional,
Slide 6.38

To summarise once more: If your child has just begun to explore its surroundings for itself it is important to remove all possible sources of danger. Then you can begin, step by step, to help your child grow up, carefully observing its development and its abilities. This process takes many years, and requires much patience. It has the best chance of success if you manage to support the spirit of discovery of your child, providing encouragement and self-confidence. This also involves paying careful attention, and it is necessary to thinks things over time and again.

Slide 6.39

Make an effort to see things through your child's eyes. Make allowances for the fact that small children have poor memories to start with, but are able to learn more and more as they grow. Respect your child's wish to do things independently and to experiment, and provide reassurance and support. Keep your eyes wide open for the objective dangers.

References

Concept for one of several slide presentations for young parents now available from the AOK Insurance Association, Kortrijker Str. 1, 53177 Bonn, Germany.

Slide presentation

Accidents in infancy

- Accidents are the most prevalent causes for **mortality in infancy.**
- The most serious accidents in infancy occur in **home and garden.**

1

Accidents in infancy

Prevention

- Provide a safe environment,
- achieve competence (parents and children)

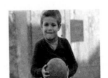

2

Slides 6.1—6.2

Accident prevention

An example
for early education
and for modeling a safe and adequate
environment for the baby.

3

Some educational principles and goals

Education is love and example,
- mediating attachment, sympathy, knowledge, skills, competence, culture,
- modeling the social interaction and the home environment,
- setting limits.

4

Slides 6.3—6.4

Accidents in infancy

- In the first two years of life an unsafe and unsecured home is as dangerous as a mine field.

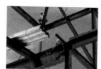

5

Accidents in infancy
Environmental risks I

Falls
- from baby's drawer,
- out of crib,
- from chair, desk, sofa,
- from high chair,
- out of window,
- from stairs,
- from balcony.

6

Slides 6.5−6.6

Accidents in infancy
Environmental risks II

Injuries by

- Falling objects,
- household tools,
- knifes, scisors, needles, pins, weapons,
- sharp edges,
- slipping carpets and mats,
- littered objects (stumbling over),
- glas doors.

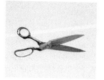

7

Accidents in infancy
Environmental risks III

Burns, scalds

- Baby in your arm, hot object in your hand,
- hot pots at the brim of stoves and tables,
- unsecured furnace,
- tap water too hot,
- burning candle,
- open fire in the living area.

8

Slides 6.7−6.8

Accidents in infancy
Environmental risks IV

Poisoning, aspiration

- Small objects,
- hard lumps of food, e.g. peanuts and carrots,
- medicine, household chemicals, sprays,
- cleaning agents, shoeblack,
- fertilizers, herbicides,
- unlocked drawers and cupboards.

9

Accidents in infancy
Environmental risks V

Traffic

- Rude **driving**,
- even short **inattentiveness**,
- inadequate **security** measures (e.g. belts),
- stay at entrance of **garage**,
- in **streets**,
- in **parking lots**.

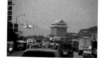

10

Slides 6.9−6.10

Accidents in infancy
Environmental risks VI

Drowning in
- swimming pools,
- water buckets,
- water toilet,
- bath tubs with more than 10 cm of water,
- puddles.
- Attention: water poisoning by baby swimming (swallowing water)!

11

Accidents in infancy
Personality risks

Infants
- are very **courious**,
- are always in **motion**,
- are naive and **do not know dangers**,
- are **clumsy**,
- have a poor sense of **balance**,
- have a **short memory** and
- and have an **egocentric view of life**.

12

Slides 6.11−6.12

Age 6 to 12 months
New skills - new risks

Expanding roaming area:

- Recognising **distant** objects.
- Developing **ability to move:**
  turn, roll, creep, crawl, pull, stand, walk.

13

Age 6 to 12 months
New skills - new risks
Going and exploring faster

- **Walk,**
- **run,**
- **climb,**
- **open container,**
- **pull drawer,**
- **switch and turn button.**

14

Slides 6.13−6.14

Risky situations
Family problems

- Overtired, **exhausted parents**,
- argumenting parents,
- **move** of home,
- stressing **life events**,
- occupational **stress**,
- **visits, journeys**,
- **babysitting**.

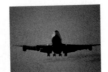

15

Checklist for a safe environment I

- Medicine, cleaning agents etc. have a **childproof** lid and seal, they are locked away,
- **cigarettes and alcohol** are out of reach,
- the phone-number of the **poison control center** is visible and well known (e.g. Berlin: 030-19240),
- **charcoal** and defoaming medicine held in readiness,
- **nuts, pearls, buttons, button batteries** are put away,
- there are no **poisonous plants** in house and garden.

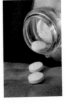

16

Slides 6.15−6.16

Checklist for a safe environment II

- The temperature of hot tap water is kept at less than **50 °C,**
- **hot beverages,** food, stove, oven, furnace and other objects are secured and out of reach,
- handles of pots and pans are **turned away**
- **matches** are kept away
- **smoke detector and fire exhauster** are in every area.

17

Checklist for a safe environment III

- **Baby walkers** are **not** used,
- the **mattress** of the baby crib is lowered,
- windows are **secured** against opening,
- **scissor fences** are **never** used to shut off stairways and rooms,
- the **high chair** cannot tip over, the infant is wearing a **belt,**
- **sharp objects** are out of reach of the infant,
- **edges** of furniture are rounded,
- the **floor** is soft (e.g. carpet ed),
- **stairs** cannot be reached without help.

18

Slides 6.17−6.18

Checklist for a safe environment IV

- The baby wears a **safety belt** in the stroller,
- only age-adjusted child **safety seats** are used in the car,
- attention is paid to the **airbag** problem,
- even for short distances a **safety belt** is used in the car,
- the baby cannot move into a **street,**
- he never plays close to a **garage.**

19

Checklist for a safe environment V

- **Drawers** filled with sharp and dangerous objects are blocked,
- **a table cloth** is not used,
- **glasses and bottles** are unreachable,
- the infant cannot get hold of a **plastic bag** or envelop,
- **cords and ropes** are not used (risk of strangulation)
- the **pacifier** is not corded,
- **pets** are banned from the infant's room.

20

Slides 6.19−6.20

Checklist for a safe environment VI

- **Electric cords** cannot be reached,
- **wall sockets** are secured,
- plug contacts and connectors are **pulled.**

21

Checklist for a safe environment VII

- Open waters of more than **10 cm** depth (buck, pail, water toilet, bathroom) are unreachable,
- the swimming pool, and the garden pond is **fenced,**
- the bottom of the bath tub is made **unslippery.**

22

Slides 6.21−6.22

Checklist for a safe environment VIII

- The infant is **never** left **alone** in the bath tub,
- he cannot **lock** himself inside the **bath room,**
- **puddles** are watched with suspicion,
- baby swimming is avoided.

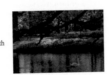

23

Protective environmental factors I

Well organized conditions:
- reliable **employment** of the main family provider,
- stable **economic** situation,
- **sufficient cash** for the required safety installations in the home.

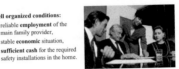

24

Slides 6.23–6.24

Protective environmental factors II

- **Well-ordered home,**
- **well-known persons,**
- having **time for the infant,**
- **no hectically** organized activities.

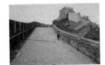

25

Protective family factors I

- Caring persons are **knowledgeable** in infant development,
- they **include** the infant competent into their lifes,
- mother, father and other caretakers **support** each other,
- they can **understand and learn,**
- they are **actively** organizing their task.

26

Slides 6.25–6.26

Protective family factors II

- They are relaxed and **concentrated,**
- they developed a secure mutual and infant **bonding,**
- the climate is kind, optimistic and **supportive,**
- they consider their role as meaningful and **manageable.**

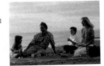

27

Age 6 to 12 months
Protective personality factors I

Infants at this age
- are eager and **able** to learn,
- like to be **praised,**
- are **willing** and benign,
- **cling** to their parents or caring persons,
- develop a **fear of strange,**
- are light, elastic and well-**cuhioned,**
- have a good **healing** capacity for injuries.

28

Slides 6.27–6.28

Age 6 to 12 months
Protective personality factors II

Infants at this age
- enlarge their **visual field,**
- improve their **perceptive capacity,**
- aquire more **physical control** over their body
- develop **manual skills,**
- improve their **memory span**
- store **experiences,**
- develop **verbal comprehension** abilities.

29

Age 6 to 12 month
They learn by perception

- Observing,
- feeling,
- feeling pain,
- licking,

- tasting,
- smelling,
- listening,
- perceiving.

30

Slides 6.29–6.30

Age 6 to 12 months
They learn by doing

- Grasping, handling,
- tasting, mouthing,
- making disappear,
- searching,
- imitating,

- repeating,
- making noise,
- exploring the environment,
- triggering reactions,
- physically exercising.

31

Promotion of Development

- **Create a safe area** for the infant allowing him to **train and explore,**
- Have a **cordial and trustful relation** to your infant,
- **Play and interact** with your infant,
- Talk to him, sing and dance with him,
- Give him faszinating **toys** for looking, feeling, smelling, rattling, building, constructing, puzzling etc.,
- Respect and promote his **independence,**
- Support his natural **learning** drive.

32

Slides 6.31–6.32

Toys (from 8 months) I
Unbreakable - washeable- not too small

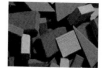

- For mind, heart and hands

Cups, bowls, pails, boxes, unbreakble mirrors, toys for the bath tub building blocks of differing shape play box big dolls, teddies, cars

33

Toys (from 8 months) II

For mind, heart, and hands...

- Picture books with large, simple pictures (cardboard, fabric, plastic)
- Toy telephone
- Cardboard tubes, boxes, egg boxes, finished magazines, plastic bottles

34

Slides 6.33–6.34

Toys (from 8 months) III

To train balance, co-ordination and orientation
- Body of the parents,
- Things to push,
- Movable objects, e.g. balls, rolls..,
- Things to pull,
- Stairs, scaffoldings, slides - under assistence,
- Toy houses with windows,
- Various types of seats.

35

Good Sources of Information I
(in Germany)

- Bundeszentrale für gesundheitliche Aufklärung (BZgA)
  Postfach 910152. 51071 Köln:
  Sicherheitsfibel - Ratgeber für Eltern zur Verhütung von Kinderunfällen
- Arbeitsausschuss Kinderspiel und Spielzeug
  Heimstraße 13, 89073 Ulm: Testmarke Spielgut
- Deutsches Institut für Normung
  Beuthverlag GmbH, 10772 Berlin, Tel. 030-26010

36

Slides 6.35–6.36

Good Sources of Information I
(in Germany)

- Erste Hilfe. Unfälle mit Kindern.
  Bundesarbeitsgemeinschaft Kindersicherheit - Safe Kids.
  Bundesvereinigung für Gesundheit e.V.,
  Heilsbachstraße 30, 53123 Bonn
- Anleitung zur Prävention von Kinderunfällen. Deutsches Grünes Kreuz. Schuhmarkt 4, 35037 Marburg/Lahn
- SP Shelov, RE Hannemann:
  Caring for your baby and young child.
  American Academy of Pediatrics. Oxford University Press, 1997

37

The safe introduction into the risky and beautiful world of adults I

- **At the beginning,**
  all potential risks need to be excluded,
  all "mines" must be defused or removed,
- **Then,**
  observe the developmental progress, and introduce your child step by step into the world of the grown-ups.
- **The process**
  takes many years, requires much of your patience, understanding, encouragement, great alertness, and consideration.

38

Slides 6.37–6.38

The safe introduction into the risky and beautiful world of adults II

Take into account
- The views and visual field of your child,
- his slowly increasing memory and ability to learn,
- his desire to act on his own,
- having fun experimenting,
- his increasing need for independence,
- his desire for appreciation, and encouragement,
- his naivity, and benignity,
- the objective risks.

39

Slides 6.39

7 "Growing up safely": a campaign promoting child safety at home

Gerald Furian, Michaela Gruber

7.1 Introduction

The Growing up Safely programme ("*Sicher gross werden*") is an Austrian model educational campaign with the aim of making young parents with small children more aware of accident prevention issues.

The programme is based on the fact that encouraging people to behave more safely can only have limited impact. It is impossible to be on permanent guard regarding potential sources of danger. Passive measures tend to have a much more reliable and longer-lasting effect by eliminating or ameliorating specific dangers so that human carelessness does not have painful, or even tragic, consequences.

If such measures are to be implemented and accepted by the public, adequate education and information will be necessary to increase awareness of safety issues and accident prevention.

7.2 Background

In Europe, accidents are the most common cause of death in children. As a consequence, accident prevention is one of the primary public health issues, and the EU member states were encouraged to make accident prevention a public health priority. The most relevant objectives defined by the WHO "Health 2000" document for Europe include a 25 % reduction in fatal and a 10 % reduction in non-fatal accidents.

Most accidents involving children are avoidable. However, if accidents involving young children are to be avoided, early parental information is necessary. This requires an educational campaign involving the help of birth clinics and parent advisory centres, so that the maximum number of parents with young children can be informed about typical accident risks in the home.

7.2.1 The research study "Home, Leisure and Sports Accidents Involving Children", and the Accident Recording System, EHLASS

The above mentioned study provided an overview of the frequency, circumstances and causes of accidents involving children at home or during leisure and sporting activities (in Austria). The relevant surveys were carried out in 1991. The evaluation of the results was completed in 1992, and a report was produced the same year. The study was carried out according to the hospital survey model and was based on a sample of 21 Austrian hospitals. Extrapolation of the results for 1991 gave an esti-mated total of 200 000 home, leisure and sporting accidents involving children and requiring subsequent hospital treatment in Austria.

The European Home and Leisure Accident Surveillance System – EHLASS – pro-vides more recent data on accidents involving children. This system is also used in Austria, and supervised by the *Institut "Sicher Leben"*, and is supported by the European Commission.

Accident patterns involving children at home were analysed using these data sources; the results were used as a background for planning the "Growing up safely" pro-gramme.

7.2.2 Accidents at home

Each year in Austria, there are approximately 90 000 accidents at home involving children under the age of 15 (i. e. 64 accidents per 1000 children). About 1 000 of these children suffer some kind of permanent injury, and more than 50 are killed. Around 52 000 (58 %) of these accidents happen to children under the age of seven. This means that every day in Austria about 140 small children are involved in an accident at home – with a fatal accident occurring statistically every two weeks (there are about 30 fatal accidents each year).

Falls are the most common form of accident (35 %), followed by collision with an object (24 %). These accidents usually occur while the child is walking, running or crawling around at home.

Another 24 % of accidents involve children being cut, pierced, caught in doors etc. These accidents occur most frequently when children are playing, 'experimenting' or are around household appliances or DIY equipment.

Burns and scalds (6 %) are typical accidents for children during their first 3 years of life. Such accidents occur mainly around ovens, furnaces, cooking surfaces, dinner tables or in the bath.

Intoxications account for about 3 % of accidents, mostly involving small children. Crawlers and toddlers tend to explore their surroundings with their mouths. Over 50 % of intoxications are due to medicine or tobacco products.

7.3 Objectives

Young children are most likely to suffer accidents at home. Many of these accidents could be avoided if young parents took appropriate preventive measures at an early stage.

The main aim within the "Growing Up Safely" programme was to use the media to inform as many young parents as possible in German-speaking countries about typical accident risks at home and ways to avoid them. This way, parents' understanding of safety issues as well as safety standards for young children could be improved.

The "Growing Up Safely" programme also served as a model for an educational campaign which could be integrated into perinatal parental health education schemes. The design of the model was flexible enough for an adaptation to the individual problems and needs of other member countries of the European Union.

7.4   Project partners

7.4.1 INSTITUT "SICHER LEBEN"

The "Institut Sicher Leben" (literally: "live safely") is part of the Austrian Safety and Prevention Board ("Kuratorium für Schutz und Sicherheit") and deals with accident research and prevention at home and during leisure or sports activities. A key component of the work of the institute is the prevention of accidents involving children. In cooperation with the Austrian Consumers' Association ("Verein für Konsumenteninformation"), the "Institut Sicher Leben" submitted the "Growing Up Safely Project" to DG XXIV of the EU, received funding approval, and managed the project through to completion.

7.4.2 VEREIN FÜR KONSUMENTENINFORMATION/STIFTUNG WARENTEST

The "Verein für Konsumenteninformation" (VKI) (Austrian Consumers' Association) is a non-profit organisation representing consumers' interests by monitoring and publishing the quality of consumer goods and providing services for Austrian consumers, and by supplying consumers with legal information and support. The VKI provides a wide range of services, including telephone advice lines, personal advisory sessions and various informative publications including the monthly consumer magazine "Konsument". This magazine features product tests, reports, and an "Extra Service" designed to be of practical help to the consumer. Special issues on specific problems (such as child safety) are also published under the title "Konsument extra". The German partner organization of the VKI, "Stiftung Warentest" publishes the monthly consumer magazine "test".

7.4.3 THE AUSTRIAN "BUNDESMINISTERIUM FÜR UMWELT, JUGEND UND FAMILIE"

The Austrian Ministry for Environmental Protection, Youth, and Family Affairs (Bundesministerium für Umwelt, Jugend und Familie) — Department IV/4 (General Family Affairs) — also participated in the "Growing Up Safely" programme.

7.5   Components of the programme

7.5.1 The Model House: "Child-Safe House"

The model house is designed like a doll house and makes an attractive wall display for birth clinics or parent advisory centres. The display shows common accident risks at home and important child-safety products (including protection for cooking and heating appliances, window locks and smoke detectors). Information leaflets can be taken from a dispenser next to the display.

7.5.2 The "Growing Up Safely" brochure

The brochure provides information about products commonly used to reduce the risks of accidents to young children in the home.

7.5.3 The Giraffe poster

The "Giraffe" poster includes a measuring scale on which the child's growth can be marked, and is an ideal decoration for a child's room. It also shows information on the developmental stages of a young child and the accident risks associated with each stage. The poster was distributed through so-called "baby packages" provided by local councils, regional governments, birth clinics and parent advisory centres.

7.5.4 Konsument Extra/Test Spezial: "Living With Children — Growing up Safely"

Special issues of "Konsument" and "test" were also published which included a comprehensive description of how to furnish and design a home with regard to the safety of small children. In 1997, the publications were mailed to around 90 000 parents in Austria and Germany; they are also available at book and newspaper shops.

7.5.5 The "Giant Kitchen" exhibition stand

The so-called "giant kitchen" was exhibited at every public presentation of the "Growing Up Safely" programme. This oversized kitchen model allows parents to experience a kitchen from the point of view of a small child, giving them a better understanding of the risks posed by standard household objects such as saucepans, knives, or bottles of cleaning fluid.

7.5.6 Courses, training programmes, and a material package

The "Growing Up Safely" course, like the "Konsument extra" special issue, also informs about designing and furnishing a home with child safety in mind. A materials package has been developed for a course of this kind, including the text of the oral presentation, background information, overhead sheets with illustrations, instructions for group activities and lists of suppliers. The course is designed to meet the requirements of antenatal parent information programmes held in parent advisory centres and birth clinics. Another course was also developed to train tutors in parent information programmes. In addition to the course, the teachers receive the material package they can use for their own teaching activities. A pilot version of this training course has already been tested in Vienna, in preparation for nationwide application.

7.6 Approach

With the approval of the Austrian Ministry of Environment, Youth and Family Affairs, all regional authorities were invited to participate in the programme.

The regional governments were given the option of selecting elements of the programme suiting the existing infrastructure in their region (for example, not all regions offer parents a "baby package"). As a result, not all regional governments participated in the programme to the same degree. Instead, individual regional approaches were developed and implemented.

For most of the regions taking part, the "Growing Up Safely" programme is the beginning of a long-term co-operation between Institut "Sicher Leben" and the birth clinics, parent advisory centres and possibly other contact points for parents (e. g. paediatricians).

In Germany, the programme focused on the distribution of the "test" special issue, "Living with children – growing-up safely".

7.7 Evaluation

A pilot project was carried out between October 1997 and the end of April, 1998; the project was monitored through a concurrent evaluation project.

7.7.1 Results of the Evaluation

The main objective of the accompanying evaluation study was to evaluate the impact of the pilot campaign on the awareness, attitude and behaviour of respondents. Media studies showed that the campaign was basically successful in reaching the target audience. The additional material was appreciated and widely used by parents. Knowledge of safety products increased significantly (+21%) and parents also felt much better informed regarding child safety at the end of the pilot project (+14%). A significant growth in the use of safety products was observed, although the increase was not as great as that for product awareness (+10%).

7.8 Conclusions

The investigation showed that even relatively short-term measures can be successful. The first stage target of the programme (an increase in public awareness of child accident prevention) was certainly achieved. Of course, if current communication activities are not continued at the same level, a slow reduction in child safety awareness is likely. If sustainable benefits are to be achieved, long-term programmes will be necessary. Therefore, it will be at least recommendable to continue the activities, and additional efforts should be made to extend the campaign to other media.

Responsible institutions should also ensure that passive accident prevention measures become a standard part of their activities and are not left to single campaigns.

7.9 Expansion of the programme since the pilot project

Recently, paediatricians were included in the campaign, so that every paediatrician in Austria has free access to project materials.

The information video "Hello, here I am − safe and sound!" was developed in co-operation with the Association of Austrian Social Security Institutions. The video is intended for viewing in paediatricians' waiting rooms and in birth clinics. Parents can also order the video for private use at home.

"Sicher Leben" has also influenced building regulations and made suggestions for regional governments on how these regulations (including support policies and guidelines on fittings and fixtures) might be modified to improve child safety. This work is supported by the Consumer Protection Minister of Austria.

7.10 References

[1] Furian, G., Gruber, M. (1998). Evaluation der Aktion "Sicher gross werden". Vienna: Institut "Sicher Leben".

[2] Media Market Observer (MMO) (1998). Effizienzmessung "Institut Sicher Leben". Analyse der Presseberichte der Aktionen "Sicher gross werden" und "Kindersicherheit zu Hause". Unpublished internal report.

[3] Schlintl, E., Goethals, B. (1992). Kinderunfälle in Haushalt, Freizeit, Sport: Ergebnisse einer österreichweiten Studie. Vienna: Literas, 2nd Ed.

[4] Sicher Leben (1998). EHLASS Austria Annual Report 1997. Vienna: Institut "Sicher Leben".

[5] World Health Organization (WHO) (1993). Ziele zur "Gesundheit für alle". Die Gesundheitspolitik für Europa. Copenhagen: WHO Regional Office for Europe.

8 Prevention of childhood injuries in Germany

Inke Schmidt, Uwe Prümel-Philippsen

8.1 Introduction

Accidents are usually associated with terms such as bad luck, fate, carelessness, and misfortune. For the victims, accidents are generally confusing and incomprehensible. In fact though, as with medical illnesses, there are many risk factors which can favour the occurrence of an "accident" event, or which, if sufficient attention is paid to them can help to prevent such an event. To this extent, measures to prevent accidents can be of key importance for the promotion and protection of health, and therefore for health itself.

In addition to traffic accidents, the most common types are accidents at work, at home and during leisure activities. Since there is no uniform registration of data for the various accident categories, the statistics presented here has been collated from various sources, which use differing assessment criteria.

8.2 Why are accidents relevant for health promotion?

In Germany, as in other industrialised nations, accidents represent the most important risk factor affecting children's health. More children older than 12 months die as a result of accidents in Germany (715 in 1997) than from infectious illnesses (122) and cancer (357) together (German Federal Statistics Office, 1999).

According to calculations of the Federal Agency for Work Safety and Medicine (BAuA), in 1995 some 8.61 million people in Germany were involved in accidents. This included more than 2 million children (Fig. 8.1). Accidents are the second most common reason after respiratory illnesses for children to be presented to a doctor.

More boys are involved in accidents than girls (approximately 60:40).

A large proportion of accidents take place at school (43%) and at home (22%) and during leisure and play (18.4%).

Typical accidents are caused by falling over while moving, falling down while climbing or falling off bicycles etc., as well as accidents with appliances and machinery,

Accidents involving children 1996

13.2 m	No. of children in Germany
>2 m	Total no. of accidents involving children
1400	Resulting in permanent disability (WHO)
774	Fatalities
1 065 000	Accidents in school
230 000	Traffic accidents
614 000	Domestic and leisure accidents of which
334 000	at home
190 000	in leisure time and play
90 000	sport

Fig. 8.1: Accidents involving children (1996)

Fatal accidents with children 1997

	0–1	1–5	5–10	10–15	Total
Poisoning		4	3	4	11
Falls	6	18	12	8	44
Burns	3	29	19	4	55
Drowning	5	56	51	13	125
Suffocation	38	26	10	11	85
Electrocution		4	3	4	11
Road traffic	16	81	102	106	305
Railways		2	2	6	10
Others	4	24	20	21	69
Total (E800–E949)	72	244	222	177	715

Fig. 8.2: Fatal accidents with children 1997

but there are also accidents which more frequently have serious consequences, such as road accidents, drowning, burns and scalds or poisoning (Fig. 8.2).

8.3 Investigating causes

The causes of many accidents involving children are related to their stage of development. Further causes can be the personality structure of the child, an insecure environment, and also additional social factors.

8.3.1 Age-specific development

In general, children have not yet developed a full awareness of dangers. For examples, it is only when they reach the age of about 8–9 years old that they are able to judge heights, distances, and speeds correctly. Children are not yet able to anticipate what other people will do in many situations. They can easily be distracted, but on the other hand if they are immersed in play, or some other activity, they are not able to maintain awareness for other things at the same time. They want to try everything out, they are inquisitive, they have a thirst for knowledge and action.

Even when the children have fully developed the above abilities, they are still very often unable to judge their own limitations. In particular boys frequently overestimate what they are capable of (Limbourg, 1998).

Adolescents tend to seek out danger and they feel an urge to take things to the limit. They seek out and provoke challenges, competitions, and risky situations. They learn complicated sequences of movements very quickly, have very sharp reactions, and good mobility and flexibility. They are attracted to fast sports which place high demands on coordination, like skateboarding, snowboarding, inline-skating or mountain biking.

8.3.2 Personality structure

In addition to traits that are frequently associated with a certain level of development of the child, there are also individual features that are relevant for accident risks. Köhler (1997) was able to establish a number of personality characteristics associated with an increased risk of accidents. Extroversion, sociability, freedom from anxiety, experience orientation, or self-overestimation, in combination with limited self-control and self-reflection are typical for children at increased risk of having accidents – in particular when several of these characteristics come together (see also Schlag and Schupp in this book).

8.3.3 Environmental factors

In addition to the factors already mentioned, there are a number of factors related to the environment and surroundings of children which also play an important role in their involvement in accidents. In particular, these can include urban and traffic planning measures, the design of buildings, playgrounds, and sports facilities, the safety of products and the care and responsibility of adults towards children (Limbourg, 1994).

8.3.4 Social factors

Social factors can also play a role when children are involved in accidents. Children from single parent families, from ethnic minorities, or from families with a low socio-economic status have a higher risk of being involved in an accident (Oerter et al., 1987; Oppolzer, 1986). Special risks may be a home that is not safe for children, for example with unprotected stairways or balconies, or unsafe electrical fittings. Unhindered access to cleaning agents, chemicals, medical supplies, and tools can also lead to accidents. In a study of accident-related hospital stays in relation to social status there was a marked over-representation of the lowest vocational status group. The difference in ages of the accident-victims was particularly marked. Whether the reason for this discrepancy lies in the layout of the accommodation, in its location, the lack of adequate supervision, or other factors remains to be determined (*Geyer*, 1998).

8.4 Accident prevention

Experts estimate that some 60% of accidents could be prevented by the enforcement of legislation, the implementation of technical measures (engineering), and by educational measures and training (Fig. 8.3).

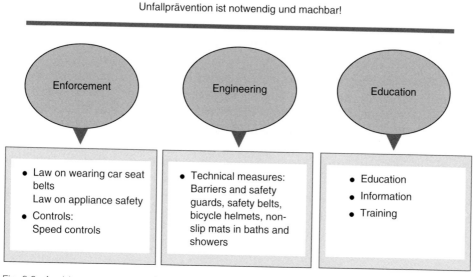

Fig. 8.3: Accident prevention

8.4.1 Legal measures, standards, and regulations (Enforcement)

Legal measures can have far-reaching consequences for human safety and for the effects of accidents. Positive examples are work safety provisions, or the introduction of the compulsory wearing of car seat belts by children. The numbers of car accidents with fatal consequences for children decreased by 31%, and the numbers of severely injured children decreased over the same period by 21% (Pfafferott, 1998). Regular controls are necessary to ensure that legal requirements are observed (e. g. radar controls in 20 mph zones). Otherwise they will not be taken seriously and will fall into disuse. The safety of technical appliances (e. g. domestic appliances, tools, toys, sports equipment) and of commercially-used facilities are covered by the legislation on the safety of appliances. In addition, technical appliances are subjected to extensive type testing, and provided with quality marks which offer the guarantee that the tested appliance is not dangerous when used in the appropriate manner.

However, there can still be problems when appliances are used by children, because they may often be unaware of the correct mode of application, and may use an appliance in a way that can be very dangerous, and even life-threatening. Therefore security experts are demanding stricter test criteria or an additional test for "Child Safety" of products, so that there is no danger even if the appliance is not used in the intended manner (German Health Association, 1995).

8.4.2 Technical measures (Engineering)

Technical measures for accident prevention include all active and passive measures that can lead to increased safety. For every age group and in all areas of life, measures are adopted such as passive safety precautions, for example protective rails, doors, safety clothing, special floor surfaces, safety belts, airbags etc. Many of these measures are required by law. But in every household there are many other dangers (especially for children!) which can be avoided relatively simply. It is estimated that some 70% of existing safety problems for children could be eliminated by technical measures (Hugi, 1995). Experts complain that towns, residential areas, houses, apartments, gardens, roads, playgrounds, vehicles, household appliances, furniture, etc., ignore the needs of children, and are still constructed so that an imminent danger to children cannot be excluded (Henter, 1997; Gruber, 1995; Schimpl et al., 1995). But adults, too, can be protected against injuries, for example by wearing bicycle helmets, or can avoid typical domestic injuries, for example by having non-slip mats in baths and showers.

8.4.3 Education, training and information

The goal of educational measures and information campaigns is to increase awareness about "Safety" and "Accident prevention". Everybody should know how their actions can influence their safety and the safety of others. People should be able to recognise dangers, to assess them, and to cope with them or avoid them all together, as well as learning about how to eliminate them at the earliest possible stage. Target groups for such awareness-raising measures include in particular people who have responsibility for others, such as parents, teachers, politicians, planners, etc. Training measures, consisting of both theoretical and practical elements, are intended to increase the ability to cope with dangerous situations. Appropriate behaviour and responses can be trained, and participants can learn to recognise dangers sooner and to avoid them, as well as course as learning how to help effectively in emergencies.

8.5 Accident prevention in Germany

In Germany there are a variety of institutions that are involved in accident prevention and have responsibility for the implementation of preventive measures, and some key institutions are shown in Figure 8.4.

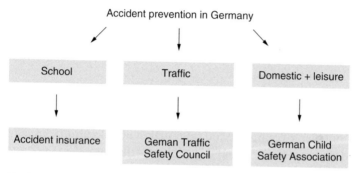

Fig. 8.4: Key institutions involved in accident prevention in Germany

8.5.1 Preventing traffic accidents

Measures to prevent traffic accidents are coordinated by the German Traffic Safety Council (DVR), the umbrella organisation for all the institutions that are involved in aspects of traffic safety. By means of campaigns and specially targeted programmes (learner drivers, older people, children, motor-bike riders, etc.) they increase awareness about particularly dangerous behaviour on the roads, in order to promote the sense of responsibility and the willingness to make special allowances for others.

As an example, since 1980 the DVR has been providing the programme "Children and Traffic", an educational programme for parents. It consists of a number of modules, for example the child as pedestrian, the child as cycle rider, or the child as passenger. The parents are informed about the abilities and limitations of small pedestrians, cycle riders, etc., and they are shown what contributions they can make to help their children become safe and independent as they move about in traffic (Fig. 8.5).

The programme has proved successful: the numbers of children killed on the roads has fallen from 1159 for the former West Germany alone in 1980, to 311 in 1997 for

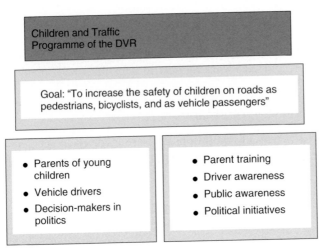

Fig. 8.5: Programm Children and Traffic (DVR)

the entire united Germany. This success was achieved despite the fact that traffic densities almost doubled over this period, although it should also be noted that the numbers of children in each age group declined over this period too (*German Child Safety Association* 1998).

8.5.2 Prevention of school accidents

All children attending play-schools, schools and higher education institutions are automatically covered by an official accident insurance scheme, which covers the effects of any accident that takes place in the educational institution, as well as on the way there and back home again.

The insurance bodies have the responsibility to ensure by all appropriate means that accidents and threats to health are avoided, as well as providing for necessary rehabilitation measures and compensation for accident victims.

The school has an important role to play in accident prevention. Firstly, most accidents involving children take place at school, and secondly it is an important location for the socialisation of children. The accident insurance agencies have therefore produced a wide range of information materials − including guidelines and security regulations, as well as brochures, teaching materials, posters, and information films. The work for increased safety in school is not restricted to avoiding accidents in connection with the school visit, but is also hoped to lead to benefits in all areas, including the journeys to and from school, at home and during recreation, as well as in the preparation for future working life.

8.5.3 Prevention of domestic and leisure accidents

For a long time there was no single institution in Germany responsible specifically for matters relating to accidents suffered by children at home and during leisure activities. After a long period of preparation, the German Association for Health, acting on behalf of the Health Ministry, came together in 1997 with 18 other institutions involved in preventing accidents to start up the campaign "More Safety for Children − Safe Kids". The participating institutions have joined together to form the German Working Association for Child Safety and have set themselves the goal of improving the coordination and cooperation between the bodies working in the field of prevention of accidents to children, with the aim of reducing the frequency of accidents involving children − in particular at home and during leisure activities − and also to reduce their severity.

The campaign "More Safety for Children" has the following goals:

- To act as advocate for the interests of children in order to avoid accidents and increase safety
- To improve product safety
- To reduce the number and severity of falls by the early development of movement skills by children
- To reduce the numbers of accidents involving drowning, falls, poisoning, and suffocation by making parents and those in charge of children more aware of problems and dangers involved
- To address the special problems faced by socially-disadvantaged parts of the population

In order to achieve these goals, four working groups were set up: Practical measures for accident prevention; Strategic measures for accident prevention; Evaluation, statistics and health reporting; Product safety. These working groups then each developed their own strategies.

The following specific measures have been or are currently being implemented:

- Annual priority 2000 of BAG: Prevention of fall injuries
- Provision of funds for project partners to carry out projects related to the BAG's annual priority; e. g. further training for play-school personnel, parent seminars, surveys
- First German Child Safety Day of the BAG with a central launch in May 2000 and various regional events under the slogan: "Watch out − Dangers!"
- Poster for all member institutions "2 million children involved in accidents in Germany every year is too many − We are doing something!" with space to announce activities

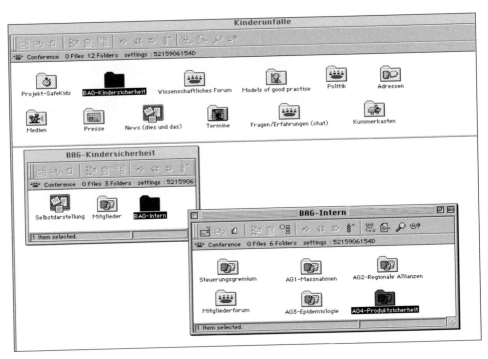

Fig. 8.6: BAG website on child safety

- BAG website on child safety: www.kindersicherheit.de (Fig. 8.6)
- Intranet forums on selected topics relating to child safety with members of BAG and key figures (Fig. 8.7)
- First-aid brochures about accidents in the home and during leisure time
- Special features on "Child safety" in the free quarterly magazine "*Kind & Gesundheit*" (Child and Health) distributed by family doctors
- Participation in the REWE-Happy Family Days promotion
- Lectures and PR work

These measures within the framework of the campaign "More Safety for Children – Safe Kids" are a first step towards increasing awareness for the topic of accident prevention among children themselves, parents, and others involved with children, while at the same time also informing the general public.

The child safety working group "*BAG Kindersicherheit*" offers all those active in Germany in relation to child accident prevention with an attractive platform for the regular exchange of information, as well as for cooperation and quality assurance.

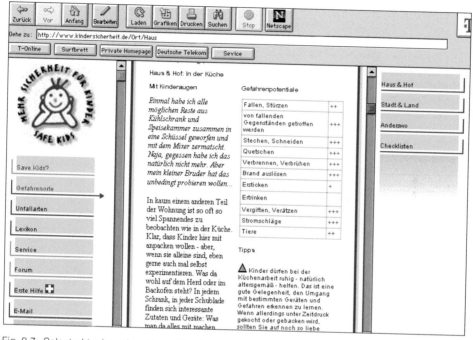

Fig. 8.7: Selected topics related to child safety on website

8.6 References

[1] Bundesanstalt für Arbeitsschutz (Ed.) 1995: Heim- und Freizeitunfälle in Deutschland. Sonderschrift p 39, Dortmund.

[2] Bundesarbeitsgemeinschaft Kindersicherheit: Pressemitteilung anlässlich der Ärztlichen Präventionstage 1998. Bonn, 21. 09. 1998.

[3] Bundesvereinigung für Gesundheit, 1995: Massnahmenkonzept zur Prävention von Kinderunfällen in Heim und Freizeit. Bonn.

[4] Geyer, S.; Peter, R., 1998: Unfallbedingte Krankenhausaufnahmen von Kindern und Jugendlichen in Abhängigkeit von ihrem sozialen Status – Befunde mit Daten ein nordrheinwestfälischen AOK. Gesundheitswesen 60, 493−499.

[5] Gruber, M., 1995: Haushalts- und Freizeitunfälle von Kindern in Österreich – ein Überblick. In: Institut Sicher Leben (Ed.): Kindersicherheit: Was wirkt? Fachbuchreihe, Vol 6, Vienna, 193−196.

[6] Henter, A., 1997: Kinder in Heim und Freizeit stark unfallgefährdet. In: Institut Sicher Leben (Ed.): Kindersicherheit: Was wirkt? Fachbuchreihe Vol 8, Vienna /Essen, 17−27.

[7] Hugi, M., 1995: Mehr Sicherheit durch Technik. In: Institut Sicher Leben (Ed.): Kindersicherheit: Was wirkt? Fachbuchreihe, Band 6, Vienna, 101−109.

[8] Köhler, G., 1997: Unfall ist kein Zufall. Psychologische Hintergründe der besonderen Unfallgefährdung des Kindes. In: Institut Sicher Leben (Ed.): Kindersicherheit: Was wirkt? Fachbuchreihe Band 8, Vienna/Essen, 291−300.

[9] Limbourg, M., 1998: Der Kinderunfall – Epidemiologie und Prävention. In: Kuratorium ZNS (ed): Tagungsbericht: Schädelhirnverletzungen bei Kindern und Jugendlichen: Prävention, Rehabilitation, Re-Integration vom 23. 10. 1997 in Düsseldorf. Bonn.

[10] Limbourg, M., 1994: Kinder im Straßenverkehr. GUVV, Münster.

[11] Oerter, R.; Montada, L., 1987: Moderne Entwicklungspsychologie. Munich, Psychologie Verlagsunion.

[12] Oppolzer, A., 1986: Wenn Du arm bist, mußt Du früher sterben; soziale Unterschiede in Gesundheit und Sterblichkeit. Hamburg, VSA-Verlag.

[13] Pfafferott, I.; Haas, I.: Aktuelle Zahlen und Fakten zur Sicherheit von Kindern im PKW. In: Deutscher Verkehrssicherheitsrat (Ed.): Sicherheit von Kindern im Auto. Dokumentation des Fachkongresses in Augsburg vom 15./16. Oktober 1998.

[14] Schimpl, G.; Mayr, J.; Spitzer, P.; Höllwarth, M., 1995: Spielplatzunfälle im Kindesalter. In: Institut Sicher Leben (Hrsg.): Kindersicherheit: Was wirkt? Fachbuchreihe, Band 6, Vienna, 238–260.

[15] Statistisches Bundesamt, 1999: Todesursachen in Deutschland. Wiesbaden: Metzler-Poeschel.

9 Educating young parents in first aid

Monika Vonberg

9.1 Introduction

There are several reasons why health promotion in the family in general and educating young parents in first aid especially, is of enormous importance in our society. Most of these are of social origin. In our times of small families, consisting only of three to five persons, we do not have the chance to learn from older and more experienced family members in difficult situations. We cannot rely on their advice and support in everyday life. The average family today lives on its own, and social contacts are mainly in the fields of work or leisure but seldom in everyday situations. As a consequence, we do not solve our struggles of everyday life together with a large family, but in our tiny family at home. The advisory function of the large family is now taken over by books, courses, health magazines and when we are ill, by doctors. When we are seriously ill for a longer period of time we are taken to hospitals and are not nursed at home by the people we know best.

Another fact is that we often try to put aside difficult situations, hoping they will only happen to other people. We calm our nerves by thinking that our health system is so good, that help is available from organisations and services whenever it is urgently needed. We are accustomed to paying for every service. This gives us the feeling of being safe and frees us from personal efforts.

From this point of view the work of health organisations was and is necessary and useful. One of the most important tasks of welfare organisations is to teach first aid in order to support the emergency services in difficult situations and to enable people to help themselves. Before I come to our work with parents I would like to give a short survey of our organisation and the general review of first aid teaching in Germany in order to demonstrate the significance of our first aid programme.

9.1.1 Presentation of our organisation: Malteser Hilfsdienst

Malteser Hilfsdienst is one of five organisations in Germany operating officially as first aid associations under the Law of Civil Protection. Malteser Hilfsdienst was established in 1953 as an umbrella organisation of Deutsche Caritas; the Order of

Malta, which had its 900-year celebration in 1999, took part in the establishment.
The original goals were instructing the population in first aid and work in disaster
control. The first aid services have become one of the most important parts of our
organisation. Others include the foreign department and social services such as care,
our meals on wheels programme, visiting service as well as a youth association. The
Malteser Hilfsdienst has become a modern welfare organisation with a 900 year
tradition. We are active in all parts of Germany with about 700 departments involved, as well as more than 30 000 active first aiders and more than 800 000 sup-
porters.

9.1.2 First aid instruction in general

First aid instruction in Germany has become an important component of the society.
Three factors are essential here:

1) Since 1953 the Government has been sponsoring first aid training for the general
   public. About 600 000 people are reached by this programme annually. For 2000
   the sponsoring by the Government has been cut; in 2001 it will be completely finished.
2) Since 1969, anyone acquiring a German driving licence has to take part in a
   special training course for first aid. Here we count approximately 700 000 participants.
3) Each company is obliged to have a number of personnel trained in first aid. In
   these courses we have some 500 000 participants per annum.

At least theoretically, Austria has a significant number of people trained in first aid.
Supposing that this knowledge is available for about 3 years, there are five to six
million citizens able to give immediate assistance in emergency cases. This is about
7 percent of the total population.

But:
The majority of these participants are not volunteers but are obliged to take part in
the first aid courses. As a consequence, the motivation to assist in an emergency
case is not very great.

The programme is very general and therefore less target-group oriented and cannot
fully meet the personal interests and needs of the participants.

The instruction is aimed at the care of adults, special measures for the care of babies
or children are only rudimentary.

For these reasons, in recent years new programmes have been developed which take
into consideration the individual requirements of the participants. One of these programmes is the instruction of "First Aid for Children".

9.2 Focuses of work in our programme "First Aid for Children"

Considering the general aims of first aid organisations we see that they usually come to help people in emergency cases. This means they come to help after an incident when people need professional help. Also usually the main part of the courses in first aid for the participants is occupied by teaching measures to help people practically, in extreme cases to keep them alive. So the focus of our teaching is helping people to survive until the arrival of professional help such as ambulance and doctors.

Nevertheless, especially first aid for children courses include hints and advice concerning prevention of critical situations. Concerning the target group the Malteser Hilfsdienst is working with a partially open curriculum. This approach consists of a standard part, which includes all life-saving measures. Then the trainer can shape the remaining part of the course to suit the needs of the participants.. We determine the expectations and the main points of interest at the beginning of the courses. The teacher has a well-prepared range of topics available and is able to choose the subjects of interest from this.

The other crucial point is prevention. In principle, no emergency case is discussed without having worked out possible measures of prevention with the participants before. The range starts from the presentation of safety products to the present recommendations on vaccinations.

To give a survey of the course we present an extract of the contents:

- Behaviour towards children in emergency cases
- Definition of an emergency
- Rescue chain; i. e. general procedure/steps after an emergency case
- Different kinds of wounds
- Injuries to the face
- Burns and scalds
- Controlling of vital functions
- Loss of consciousness and recovery position
- Heatstroke, hypothermia
- Cramps, epileptic fits
- Breathing and choking, insect stings, asthma attacks
- Resuscitation
- Drowning
- Sudden infant death
- Electrical injuries
- Severe bleeding
- Shock
- Abdominal injuries
- Chemical burns and poisoning

9.2.1 The structure of teaching each topic

In order to facilitate the learning for the participants there are several steps of work in every topic:

1. visual introduction by folio or by video
2. working out preventive actions
3. theoretical background of a topic
4. identifying the emergency
5. dangers to the child
6. measures of help, practise wherever it is possible

9.2.1.1 Visual introduction by overhead projections or by video

According to the demands of being close to everyday-life and preventive concerning future situations the topics are prepared and supported by some media. So we can present overhead foils showing typical situations so that the participants can imagine the emergency. Also video clips with children in everyday situations which turn into an emergency are shown. Both media are used for several reasons:

- They introduce a new topic visually.
- They show that everyday situations can easily turn into emergencies.
- The videos also show how to react and help in the special situation.
- The videos show how to prevent some emergencies.

I would like to give a practical example to show you how the system works.

Scenario: Children are celebrating a birthday party outside. The weather is sunny, everybody is having fun. There are several children playing and some adults (mothers) are supporting the party. Some cake and sweet drinks are put on a table in glasses or cups. One child stops playing with the others and takes a drink. The child does not look into the glass, but is observing the other children.

The child drinks and the wasp stings the child in the mouth. The child starts crying, because the sting hurts and because everything in the mouth starts to swell; the child panics and finds it hard to breath.

One adult cares for the child, one calls the ambulance.

Prevention: Give the drinks in glasses with a straw. By this simple measure you avoid being stung in the mouth by insects

9.2.1.2 Working out preventive measures

One of the most important aspects of health promotion is prevention of emergencies. Although the main character of our courses is helping after an emergency has occurred, the preventive aspects is always present.

In our courses in first aid for children this does not mean long lasting measures of caring for health like for example brushing teeth to prevent caries, but it means opening the eyes for the dangers in everyday-life. People and in our case especially young parents and other people who have a lot to do with small children must realize at an early stage which dangers can occur in standard situations. This is the only chance they have to take preventive measures.

For example:

- If you give a sweet beverage to a child in summer especially when you are outside, it is better to put it in a closed cup with a drinking straw than to hand it in an open cup. If you use a straw you do not risk an insect sting in the mouth or in the throat of a child which would be very dangerous, because the child might suffocate.
- You can avoid severe wounds and injuries if you give children the chance to put their toys in low drawers in the cupboard, because they need not climb to get them.
- You must realize that small children can drown even in very shallow ponds or sometime in a tub or vat. They are not very used to keeping their balance and often fall into tubs or vats while they are playing with toys (boats, plastic ducks etc.)
- You should prevent small children from playing with plastic bags, especially when they are transparent. They often put them over their heads and can suffocate.
- You should lock electric fuses so that your child cannot get into them with the hands. Special care is necessary to explain to them that water is dangerous in contact with electricity.
- You can avoid severe burns if you do not leave small children alone with burning candles, hot ovens, hot irons etc.
- You can avoid severe scalds by putting a small guard on the cooker so that your child cannot pull at cooking pots.
- You can avoid severe injuries if you lock away your cleaning agents and try to reduce them in general to a necessary number.
- You can avoid poisoning if you lock up your medical supplies carefully.

We could name many more easy preventive measures.

Another character of prevention is to take into account the possible personal healthy defects of a child.

- If a child shows allergic reactions such as asthma attacks when it comes into contact for example with trees, flowers etc., try to keep them away from them.
- Prevention can also mean a special physical training to strengthen the heart or the muscles. In such cases medical advice and sometimes supervision is needed.

Prevention can also mean having medical supplies at home to deal with small wounds; we give our participants a list of things which they should have at home in their family first aid box.

In a wider sense prevention also means being prepared and able to help in emergency cases. In this sense our whole field of work has a preventive character. Making people ready to help in emergencies is a combination of learning theoretical background information and practising wherever possible.

9.2.1.3 Theoretical background of a topic

We teach people the theoretical basics and support their process of learning by using visual aids. By doing so, people are able to remember up to about 70 % of the subject matter. We teach them the background knowledge they need, which of course is not as much as professionals in this field.

If we take e. g. asthma attacks they learn something about normal breathing. They get information about the function of the lungs and how oxygen and carbon dioxide work in the body. They learn how often we breath at different ages and how much air is inhaled with every breath. They learn what can go wrong with breathing in general, what happens if a person does not breath at all and they learn what takes place in the body and happens when a child has an acute asthma attack. The corresponding media help the participants to memorize the contents.

9.2.1.4 Recognition signs/symptoms of the emergency

The theoretical background is interesting and necessary for the participants, but the first step is how they can realize what is wrong with their child. Therefore they must know the symptoms which occur in an emergency case. Only the knowledge of the symptoms makes people realize the situation and makes them capable of taking the right decisions. They know what to do with the child and they can decide if they must call the ambulance or take the child to a doctor.

If we continue with our asthma example, the participants learn that the child has great problems with exhaling, panics because the oxygen level in the blood is not high enough, and starts to compensate by breathing faster and faster. They try to keep or to put their body into a comfortable position, i. e. they try to sit in an upright position.

9.2.1.5 Dangers to the child

The next step is to work out the dangers to the child. Based on the theoretical background and the symptoms, the dangers to the child can be deduced. The trainer does this with the participants, so that they are involved during the whole process. Generally the degree of the dangers makes it clear to the participants that they should not lose time before starting direct help because the child is in mortal danger.

Taking the example of an asthma attack this means that the child might possibly stop breathing altogether. But the body and especially the brain needs oxygen urgently to avoid irreparable damage to the brain or even death.

So working out the dangers to the child makes it very clear to the participants that help is needed urgently. If the help is not provided the child may die.

9.2.1.6 Measures of help, practice wherever it is possible

After having laid the theoretical basis together with the participants they are open minded for the measures they must take to save the child's life. In some cases it is only possible to give them advice about what to do; in many other cases it is possible to practise the measures with them very intensively. As repetition is a decisive means of learning some actions like how to call the ambulance and how to find out if the child is unconscious, without breathing and if the heart is still beating can be repeated many times in the duration of the course.

Coming back to the asthma attack, several steps must be taken:

- Call the ambulance.
- Put the child in a comfortable position, i.e. in an upright position, propped on the hands. The child can breathe more easily.
- Calm the child down so that the panic subsides.
- Breathe together with the child; give orders when to inhale and when to exhale. Maybe you can cut the extreme frequency in this way.

Concerning the measures we can say that calming a child down and giving it the feeling of being there to help and comfort it is very important. It needs the feeling of not being alone and being helped and caressed by someone. The feeling of being cared for is a great help to calm a person down and this is in some cases very necessary for the success of other measures.

We must always keep in mind that even if the ambulance is very fast it takes about 10 to 15 minutes on average to arrive. And this is the gap which we have to bridge. It does not seem long at first sight, but in an emergency, when everybody is extremely strained 10 to 15 minutes can seem to never ending. Therefore we must be very sure in what we have to do in order to take the right decisions quickly.

9.2.2 Demands of our customers/participants

The programme is aimed at everybody in regular contact with children or babies. So parents, grandparents, teachers, kindergarten-teachers and also baby-sitters should be addressed here. These participants differ significantly from the participants of other first aid courses. While in normal courses for adults much time must be spent to overcome restraints and scruples and to motivate for assistance, participants of the courses for first aid for children have a completely different motivation. Especially young parents are characterised by an observable and clear need for safety; a possible emergency case which the course prepares for, refers directly to the own child and not some anonymous person involved in an accident.

The emotional appeal to the child is very great and this has its effects on the emotional conditions of the parents or teachers etc. They want to help the child and they know that the child's future or survival depends on them and they would have to live with the consequences of a wrong decision for the rest of their life. They would be in a stress situation and are therefore not able to think logically. So they must have a well-known pattern of action which they can follow. This is crucial especially for the beginning of the action.

So the main demand of our customers is to equip them to take the right decisions, supplying them with a strategy of action and making them fit in practical measures. For them, prevention means being prepared for the emergency case and being open-minded for realising dangers in advance and to take several precautionary measures so that the dangerous situations of everyday-life can be avoided completely or at least be minimised.

Additionally they would like to learn more about tending to so-called trifle injuries such as knee wounds etc.

But the requests of the participants about daily situations seems to be very difficult in the field of medicine. The rarer situation of heart and circulatory failure of children is discussed in detail by specialists, even differentiating age groups. We are able to provide long lessons on this subject. But the topics parents actually want to know about for daily use are beyond the bounds of our possibility.

For example concerning so-called trifle injuries such as knee wounds which happen very often, we cannot do more than recommend covering the wound and seeing the doctor. However, this is neither convincing nor appropriate. Here, clear advice for practical procedure is lacking. The Help Associations are trying to solve this problem by including paediatrics as mediators. Therefore, the programme which comprises 4 units of 90 minutes each, can be extended by one more unit (90 minutes more), during which a doctor is available to answer further questions. However, there are limits on organisational and teaching capacity.

9.2.3 Our means of advertising promotion

Unfortunately, we have no sponsor for this instruction of target groups. Since at the present time the Austrian government is withdrawing from the education in first aid, the Help Associations require more support than before for this programme. Therefore free courses, such as the instruction of first aid for children, have to be financed through the participants directly. For this reason, the costs for such a course amount at present to euro 15 to 20 per participant. As a consequence, the programme only reaches those parents who are free from economic constraints, i. e. the middle class. The majority of those middle class people already have a general knowledge of prevention and first aid measures because they pay great attention to their children. However, our programme should mainly address members of the lower class who unfortunately have less time, interest and money to spend on first aid instruction. Moreover, the costs for the courses mean an additional difficulty for these people with low income, so that the future development of the programme depends on sponsors.

In some towns and cities there is co-operation with youth offices which partly pay for the instruction of their kindergarten staff.

At present the responsible trade associations together with the first aid organisations are trying to create a special course for kindergarten personnel which they are probably willing to pay for. In this case the normal contents of first aid courses for adults are filled up with special features about children.

The courses are advertised in newspapers, public places, and sometimes in local radio stations. The demand for the programme is high, especially among average parents who are by nature sensitive for health promotion, but less by the socially disadvantaged who should be led to social responsibility and awareness of health promotion.

9.3 Conclusion and demands for the future

In general, targeted courses like our first aid for children course are accepted and are in demand. The participants get practical advice about how to react and how to handle difficult emergency situations by taking the right decisions quickly and applying possibly life-saving measures.

It is very sensible to make people aware about the aspects of health promotion as early as possible. And the best chance to do so is when they have small children. But it is also necessary to accompany them in their further development so that a complete system of health promotion can be established.

From this point of view it is necessary to make even small children familiar with aspects of health promotion and to make them able and willing to help other people when they are in need. This is the only way to reach every generation in the long run.

At an early age children are not shy, they are not afraid of other people, they touch them without thinking about the possible consequences. They help without being afraid of mistakes or of contact which adults often do not like and avoid. They do not weigh costs and benefits. They help directly when they think someone needs help.

Later on people's decision in favour of or against helping depends on other preconditions, when they are not used to a sense of responsibility towards other people in difficult situations.

Winning the children means winning the parents for social aspects. We can often observe that parents come to our courses after their children were instructed in some aspects. It is a matter of pride, because the parents do not like to know less than their children. Therefore this start is a very important aspect in health promotion in general and does not only refer to emergency cases.

In order to be able to provide people with such courses, funding is necessary from the state and as far as possible from health services. The problem is not just to pay the money for the instruction of the parents. It is also very expensive to create and develop the courses and to keep the curricula up to the latest medical standards

Therefore financial support by the state and the health services is necessary to keep the courses going and to increase the number of participants who cannot pay for it by themselves.

From the medical point of view accurate standards are required to enable lay-treatment of especially minor injuries.

9.4 Discussion

Dr. Ellsässer (Chair):
... Thank you, Mrs. Vonberg, for your presentation. What I think we need, too, is a link between prevention measures and (you said) that you could implement this quite easily in (the video), and we (want) in one way what Prof. Berfenstam said: prevent those injuries, and you say, we have to inform parents in first aid: Do you think that you could link both in your organisation?

M. Vonberg:
Yes, we try to do it by giving practical examples, for example with cleaning agents, we tell people where to put them so that children do not get at them, or the example of the film was not to open the drink and put it down and then take it again, and just drink, because insects might be inside and you have the stings in your throat afterwards. In the courses, or in the instructions, the aspect of prevention takes very much space, because it is always better to prevent than to do something afterwards. And we always try to make the link.

Prof. Bergmann:
How do you think to reach a larger proportion of the population, what do you do about this?

M. Vonberg:

It is a bit difficult: In general, people phone us and call for such courses, but we also call into kindergartens and schools and offer these courses. But there is still one problem with the socially deprived groups, that we do not get them. But we also try to offer our services, and we go into schools and into kindergartens, and into groups where parents meet and things like that.

Dr. Bergmann:

Are you working together with paediatricians?

M. Vonberg:

Yes we are. In every city we have some representatives of the paediatricians, and we always try to have very close contact and try to update our programme, too, if there is new knowledge.

10 Prevention of allergy

Renate L. Bergmann, Karl E. Bergmann, Ulrich Wahn

10.1 Introduction

Allergy is already tipped to be the epidemic of the 21st century, and nearly half the population of developed countries are atopic (Johansson 2000). Atopic disease is the form of allergy that runs in families, such as atopic eczema, allergic rhinitis and asthma. These phenotypes of atopic diseases have a chronic or chronically relapsing course, and they appear from infancy in a typical chronological order, called the atopic march. The clinical symptoms are accompanied by an IgE mediated sensitisation. The first phenotypes in early infancy are atopic eczema and/or gastrointestinal symptoms, preceded or accompanied by specific antibodies against food antigens. Later on, antibodies develop against inhalative allergens and respiratory symptoms (Bergmann et al. 1994).

10.2 Etiological Factors

10.2.1 Genetics play a role

From epidemiological and genetic studies it is known that candidate genes are involved, localised for instance on chromosome 5q, 6, 11q, 16 and on chromosome X. However, environmental influences are also crucial for the expression of these diseases, gene-environment-interactions may be considered as the basis for allergic diseases (Asher et al. 2000).

10.2.2 Environmental factors

The environmental influences may be divided into the categories "protective" and "causative". Protective influences include microbial exposure, large family size, infections, dietary factors, socio-economic factors (e. g. access to medical care). Causative influences include allergen exposure to food, house dust-mite, cat, dog, vermin, environmental tobacco smoke exposure, special food ingredients, damp housing, traffic pollution, high socio-economic status, small family size (Asher 2000).

The timing of environmental exposure is important for recommendations in order to prevent the development of any atopy (primary prevention). As soon as the first symptoms and signs appear, the progress in severity or the appearance of the next atopic phenotype could be prevented (secondary prevention), while handicaps or follow-on damage should be avoided by measures for tertiary prevention.

There are many studies, including recent ones, with equivocal results on exposure in pregnancy and differing recommendations. Atopy of the mother is of major importance in programming the fetal immune system. Already at 9 weeks of pregnancy T-lymphocytes can be detected in the fetal thymus. At 14 gestational weeks B-lympho-cytes are also present in other organs, such as lung and gut, and at 19 to 20 weeks IgM-antibodies can be discovered on circulating lymphocytes, which means that the fetus is able to produce specific antibodies from the middle of pregnancy. Although peripheral mononuclear cells of the fetus are able to mount antibodies against cow's milk, egg and house dust mite from 22 weeks of gestation, prospective studies have not proved that elimination of these allergens from the diet of the expectant mother can prevent allergic sensitisation of her infant (Holt et al. 2000). More recently even a high allergy load in pregnancy has been suggested for allergy prevention. As long as there is no clear evidence for the efficiency of these methods, no preventive measures should be recommended in pregnancy apart from good nutrition and healthy living habits, including no smoking.

10.2.3 Diet

In contrast, many prospective studies have been able to prove that, after birth, elimination diets can prevent and postpone atopic disorders or ameliorate their severity in genetically predisposed children. Candidates for elimination are food components from the infant's diet or, if carefully supervised, also from the breastfeeding mother's diet, which are responsible for early sensitisation, i.e. cow's milk, egg, nuts and in some areas fish (Hattevig 1989). But, the genetic predisposition and other environmental factors will finally lead to atopic disorders in the child, although probably at an older age (Zeiger 2000). The "other factors" which seem to protect against atopic diseases, e.g. infections and microbes will hopefully be clarified in ongoing studies.

10.2.4 Infections

The allergy risk is higher for first born infants, single children, and the socially-advantaged. The risk is lower under less hygienic conditions (Strachan 1996). While early wheezing caused by viral infections is a risk factor for asthma, on the other hand frequent colds, gastrointestinal infections, measles, hepatitis A, BCG-vaccina-tion, and the early colonisation of the gut with probiotic bacteria have been shown to protect against allergies (Kalliomäki 2001). The protective role of infections is considered to be due to an early programming of T-helper (TH)-cells in the direction of TH1- rather than to TH2-functions. TH2-cells produce cytokines, which initiate the allergic reaction, while TH1-cells are involved in the defence of viral and bacterial infections and in the rejection of foreign tissues. The TH1 direction in the development of TH-cells can be stimulated even by bacterial products like lipopolysaccharides (LPS), which are plentiful in rural and agricultural areas where cattle are kept. Sensitisation against pollen and atopic rhinitis were less prevalent in children and adults who spent the first years of their life in rural areas (Leynaert 2001, Barnes 2001, Heinrich 2001). But these findings are not evidence based, so far, to serve as a basis for recommendations to prevent allergies.

10.2.5 Role of breast feeding

Another explanation for the observations in more recent follow-up studies of a higher prevalence of sensitization and asthma in school age children, adolescents and adults once breastfed, would be that breastfeeding prevented early infection associated wheezing and therefore increased the risk for later sensitization and asthma (Rusconi et al. 1999, Wright et al. 1999, 2001, Sears et al. 2002).

The epidemic spread of allergic diseases in the developed world has initiated efforts towards therapeutic intervention, preventive initiatives, and information campaigns. The enthusiasm of the doctors and the afflicted patients to spread the knowledge through the media has not diminished. This might be responsible for a secular development untying the associations observed at the beginning of the 20th century. In 1936 Grulée and Sanford observed that atopic eczema was seven times as prevalent in infants fed on cow's milk compared to breast-fed infants (Grulée and Sanford 1936, Kramer 1988). In the following decades this association could not be confirmed unequivocally. Infants of families with allergic disorders were more often breast-fed, and for longer periods, so, especially if they developed allergic symptoms this suggested the reverse causation.

The true causation could not be elucidated, because breast-feeding cannot be randomised. But a recent study by M. Kramer solved this dilemma by randomly selecting hospitals to teach personnel breast-feeding skills according to the directions of the UNICEF/WHO for baby-friendly hospitals (Kramer 2001). It turned out that the prevalence of exclusive breast-feeding of mothers attending these hospitals was significantly higher, while the eczema prevalence of their infants was significantly lower compared to the hospitals with untrained personnel.

10.2.6 Indoor allergens

The problem of indoor allergen elimination is evolving in a similar direction. While reliable studies could demonstrate that elimination of indoor allergens is a good method not only to treat patients allergic to indoor allergens, but also for primary prevention of atopic sensitisation and early respiratory symptoms; indoor allergen reduction is now a widespread recommendation for atopic families (Custovic 2001). Their home environment has far lower levels of indoor allergens and less tobacco smoke than the environment of families without atopic members (Hjern et al. 2001, Wijga 2001).

It is tempting to speculate that as soon as an indoor allergen sensitisation of the infant has been established, procedures for allergen reduction are put in place which modulate the subsequent course of the disease. This could explain why more and more studies find an association between pet ownership, a high domestic allergen load and a low prevalence of allergic diseases in families (Rönmark 2001). Tolerance induction could be an explanation. This would direct to an opposite approach for primary atopy prevention. But which allergens should be offered when, how and in what quantities are open questions.

10.2.7 Increasing prevalence and modern life style

Since allergic diseases are increasing with increasing civilisation, the idea of a causal link evolved. All the evils of the modern society seemed to turn into allergic disorders of the individuals, the unnatural, polluted environment, the artificiality of the modern world, of food processing, the genetic engineering of food-stuffs, psychological and social problems, the loss of life culture and of faith. The cure therefore was expected in the restoration of the so-called natural environment and lifestyle, the treatment of psychological and social problems, the acceptance of a surrogate faith, and a lot of voodoo. These intentions and the unequivocal recommendations of the scientific community have produced some kind of preventive nihilism. After all, can primary prevention be a goal? Should we not rather aim at secondary or even tertiary prevention?

10.3 Current recommendations

In our opinion it is the duty of all responsible doctors to avoid fear and overreaction of the people they are caring for and of the community they address. It is good to spread the knowledge of allergies, but it is also necessary to keep things in perspective. Allergic symptoms come and go, most of them are tolerable or even harmless. A calm attitude of the care-providers is the prerequisite for the application of simple procedures to ameliorate the symptoms of the child. The risks have to be explained and the doctor visited as soon as the symptoms indicate possible risks.

What are the recommendations for the prevention of atopic disorders? Although an atopic family history, and especially atopy of the mother increase the atopy risk of the infant, most infants who develop atopic disorders come from low-risk families, fig 1. Therefore primary preventive strategies should include measures from which all infants might profit, e. g. exclusive breast-feeding for 6 months, then stepwise introduction of low-allergenic solid foods, gentle cleaning and caring procedures for the skin with avoidance of allergenic products, a dust-free personal environment for the infant, avoidance of overheating by garments, bed covers or room temperature, no mould in the house, no environmental tobacco smoke, and frequent exposure to a natural environment. The pregnant mother and her infant might profit from some probiotic products.

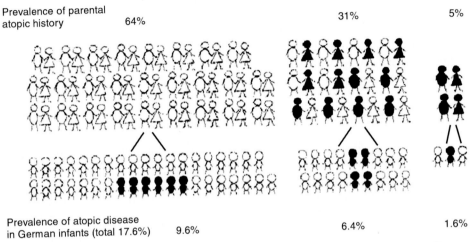

Prevalence of parental atopic history: 64%, 31%, 5%

Prevalence of atopic disease in German infants (total 17.6%): 9.6%, 6.4%, 1.6%

Fig. 10.1: Population based prevalence of atopic disease (manifestation plus sensitisation) in German infants during the first two years of life according to history of atopic disease in their parents. German Multicenter Allergy study MAS (Bergmann 1998).

As soon as sensitisation or early symptoms occur, the strategies have to be changed: Parents should become competent in the treatment of these symptoms. Good experience has been made with parent schools, i. e. group seminars for concerned parents, were teaching, practical examples, and mutual exchange produce good therapeutic outcomes. In Germany, health insurance companies support these efforts.

10.4 References

[1] Asher I, Dagli E, Holgate ST: Genetic and environmental influences. In: WHO Management of Non communicable Diseases Department: Prevention of Allergy and Asthma. WHO Interim Report. Allergy 2000; 55: 1074–1075.
[2] Barnes M, Cullinan P, Athanasaki P, MacNeill S, Hole M, Harris J, Kalogeraki S, Chatznikolaou N, Drakonakis N, Bibaki-Liakou V, Newman-Taylor AJ, Bibakis I: Crete: Does living on a farm explain urban and rural differences in atopy? Clin exp Allergy 2001; 31: 1822–1828.
[3] Bergmann RL, Bergmann KE, Wahn U: Can we predict atopic diseases using perinatal risk factors? Clin Exp Allergy 1998; 28: 905–907.
[4] Bergmann RL, Wahn U, Bergmann KE: The allergy march: from food to pollen. Envir Toxicol Pharmacol 1997; 4: 79–83.

[5] Custovic A, Simpson BM, Simpson A, Kissen P, Woodcock A and the NAC: Effect of environmental manipulation in pregnancy and early life on respiratory symptoms and atopy during first year of life: a randomised trial. Lancet 2001; 358: 188–193.

[6] Grulée CG, Sanford HN: The influence of breast and artificial feeding on infantile eczema. J. Pediatr 1936; 9: 223–225.

[7] Hattevig G, Kjellman B, Sigurs N, Bjoerksten B, Kjellman NIM: The effect of maternal avoidance of eggs, cow's milk and fish during lactation upon allergic manifestation in infants. Clin Exp Allergy 1989; 19: 27–32.

[8] Heinrich J, Gehring U, Douwes J, Koch A, Fahlbusch B, Bischof W, Wichmann HE, and the INGA-Study-group: Pets and vermin are associated with high endotoxin levels in house dust: Clin Exp Allergy 2001; 31: 1839–1845.

[9] Hjern A, Hedberg A, Haglund B, Rosén M: Does tobacco smoke prevent atopic disorders? Clin Exper Allergy 2001; 31: 908–914.

[10] Holt PG, Naspitz CK, Warner JO: Early immunological influences. In: WHO Management of Non communicable Diseases Department: Prevention of Allergy and Asthma. WHO Interim Report. Allergy 2000; 55: 1075–1077.

[11] Johansson SGO: Introduction. In: WHO Management of Noncommunicable Diseases Department: Prevention of Allergy and Asthma. WHO Interim Report. Allergy 2000; 55: 1073.

[12] Kalliomaeki A, Salminen S, Arvilommi H, Kero P, Koskinen P, Isolauri E: Probiotics in primary prevention of atopic disease: a randomised placebo-controlled trial. Lancet 2001; 1076–1079.

[13] Kramer MS, Chalmers B, Hodnett ED, and the PROBIT study group: Promotion of breastfeeding intervention trial (PROBIT). JAMA 2001; 285: 413–420.

[14] Kramer MS: Does breastfeeding help protect against atopic disease? Biology, methodology, and a golden jubilee of controversy. J Pediatr 1988; 112: 181–190.

[15] Langstein L, Rott F: Altlas der Hygiene des Saeuglings und Kleinkindes. Julius Springer Berlin 1918, Tafel 96.

[16] Leynaert B, Neukirch C, Jarvis D, Chinn S, Burney P: Does living on a farm during childhood protect against asthma, allergic rhinitis, and atopy in adulthood? Am J Respir Crit Care Med 2001; 164: 1829–1834.

[17] Roenmark E, Joensson E, Platts-Mills T, Lundbaeck B: Incidence and remission of asthma in schoolchildren: report from the obstructive lung disease in northern Sweden. Pediatrics 2001; 107: E37.

[18] Rusconi F, Galassi C, Corbo GM, Forastiere F, Biggeri A, Ciccone G, Renzoni E, and the Sidria Collaborative group: Risk factors for early, persistent, and late-onset wheezing in young children. Am J Resp Care Med 1999; 160: 1617–1622.

[19] Sears MR, Green JM, Willan AR, Taylor DR, Flannery EM, Cowan JO, Herbison GP, Pulton R: Long-term relation between breastfeeding and the development of atopy and asthma in children and young adults: a longitudinal study. Lancet 2002; 360: 901–907.

[20] Strachan D: Socio-economic factors and the development of allergy. Toxicol Letters 1996; 86: 2–3.

[21] Wijga A, Smith HA, Brunnekreef B, Gerritsen J, Kerkhof M, Koopman LP, Neijens HJ: Are children at high familial risk of developing allergy born into a low risk environment? The PIAMA Birth Cohort study, Prevention and incidence of asthma and mite allergy. Clin Exp Allergy 2001; 31: 576–581.

[22] Wright AL, Holberg CJ, Taussig LM, Martinez FD: Factors influencing the relation of infant wheezing and recurrent wheeze in childhood. Thorax 2001; 56: 192–197.

[23] Wright AL, Sherill D, Holberg CJ, Halonen M, Martinez FD: Breast-feeding, maternal IgE, and total serum IgE in childhood. J Allergy Clin Immunol 1999; 104: 589–594.

[24] Zeiger RS: Dietary aspects of food allergy prevention in infants and children. J Pediatric Gastroenterol Nut 2000; 30 (Suppl): S. 77–86.

11   Caring for the primary dentition – securing parental contributions

Svante Twetman

11.1 Introduction

Basically, erupting teeth are healthy, and the challenge for the dental profession is to help parents to keep them that way. Although a general decline in caries is evident in children from all around the world, early childhood caries (ECC) is still the major threat to oral health in infants and toddlers. ECC is a life-style disease with biological, behavioural and social determinants. Today, a vast body of evidence-based knowledge and technology is available to promote oral health and prevent caries. Even though the principles are simple and well known, it can be difficult to manage programmes for the youngest children and to get a successful contribution from the parents.

Without doubt, most effort and research has been focused on *what* to say or do rather than on *how* to say it. Furthermore, very few studies have investigated the effectiveness of various preventive strategies early in life and only limited findings are available on which kind of education and methods that really works for very young children with a high and rampant caries activity (Ismail 1998; Tinanoff et al., 1998). In the absence of reliable scientific data for this age group, preventive measures with proven efficacy in other age groups must be used. The first aim of this paper is to briefly review the ecology behind ECC and summarize suitable strategies and tools that may be used for its prevention. Secondly, with experience gained from the Public Dental Service in Sweden, some models of involving the parents or carers are suggested.

11.2 Early childhood caries – definition and epidemiology

Early childhood caries can be defined as the occurrence of any sign of dental caries on any tooth surface during the first 3 years of life. The condition has also been called nursing bottle caries, baby bottle tooth decay and nursing caries. Such terms might however be misleading since they suggest that baby bottles are always involved in the process, which is not the case. In fact, bottle use is prevalent in children both with and without caries. The prevalence of ECC varies between 1 and 12% in developed western societies (Milnes, 1996) although values up to 70%, have been reported in some native American populations, among immigrants and in underprivileged and deprived communities (Barnes et al., 1992). Most studies, however, have been cross-sectional with different diagnostic definitions and included children of various ages.

The incidence of ECC in a longitudinal whole population study was investigated among infants and toddlers in Sweden a few years ago (Wendt, 1995). The findings showed that 0.5% of the children exhibited ECC at 12 months of age, increasing to 8% at 24 months and 28% at 36 months of age. An important conclusion to be drawn from these figures is that the preventive efforts must start not later than 1 year of age. It should also be underlined that the true occurrence of ECC is difficult to establish because young children are not always cooperative for a thorough clinical examination.

In summary, the two major demographic determinants involved in ECC are ethnicity and socio-economic status. The most important variables in the former group are cultural norms, health care delivery factors and risk behaviour. A low socio-economic status including family education level, awareness and attitudes has a strong inverse relationship to the prevalence of ECC. Poor oral health often coincides with poor general health and a high risk for developmental and behavioural disorders in vulnerable and immigrant populations (Flores et al., 2002).

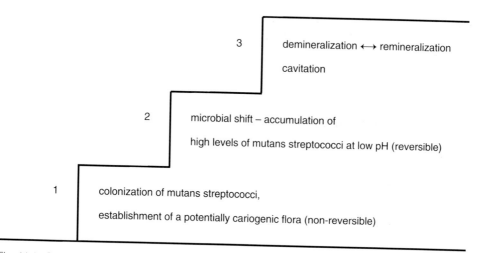

Fig. 11.1: Caries in infants and toddlers can be described as a three-step event

11.2.1 Early childhood caries – ecological aspects and clinical pattern

It is generally accepted that dental caries is an infectious and transmissible disease that is strongly modified by diet with saliva as a critical regulator (van Houte, 1994).

Caries is the result of an ecological imbalance, a disturbed homeostasis, in the oral cavity. There is evidence suggesting a three-step event in caries development as illustrated in Figure 11.1. The first step is the transmission and primary infection with mutans streptococci, a highly acidogenic and aciduric group of microorganisms. Mutans streptococci are predominantly transmitted from mothers to their infants, but recent studies using DNA fingerprinting suggest that the child may also be infected by fathers and caretakers from outside the family (Emanuelsson, 2001). The most common routes of transmission are pacifiers and spoons (Caufield et al., 1993). Mutans streptococci colonization can occur shortly after tooth eruption and high counts in mothers are associated with an early colonization of their infants (Berkowitz et al., 1981, Thorild et al., 2002).

The establishment is favoured by a sucrose-rich diet and the earlier the transmission occurs, the more caries is likely to develop in the primary dentition (Alaluusua and Renkonen, 1983; Köhler et al., 1988). Once established, the cariogenic mutans streptococci in plaque act on fermentable carbohydrates in the diet to produce even more acids. The growth of aciduric bacteria (mutans streptococci, lactobacilli, low pH non-mutans streptococci) is enhanced at the expense of less acid tolerating strains, resulting in an accumulation to pathogenic levels – a microbial shift (step 2). If left undisturbed, the low-pH environment created can demineralize the deciduous tooth enamel very rapidly (step 3). Besides, in early childhood there are several modifying etiologic factors involved that are unique for this age group. Some of them are listed in Table 11.1.

Table 11.1: Some specific factors involved in early childhood caries

microorganisms
   early colonization of mutans streptococci
   lack of oral hygiene routines

substrate
   sugar in drinks, milk and baby formulas during bedtime or naptime
   high frequency of sugar consumption from drinks and solid food
   nursing bottles, pacifiers and sucking habits
   prolonged feeding pattern

host
   low salivary flow rate at night-time
   newly erupted, immature teeth
   immature specific and non-specific defence system
   high prevalence of hypoplastic defects in primary dentition
   medical conditions

social variables
   parental education
   socioeconomic status
   siblings

Inappropriate use of the baby bottle has without a doubt a central role in the etiology and progression of ECC. The prolonged bedtime use of bottles with sweet content is especially detrimental for the young immature teeth, since the secretion of protective saliva is very low during sleep. It is also important to point out that prolonged breast-feeding on demand can be directly causative for caries. Other factors that may predispose teeth to early caries are hypomineralisation or hypoplasia (Seow, 1998). Such enamel defects are frequently reported in children born in developing countries, in disadvantaged communities of industrialized countries and in children with low birth weight. The condition is characterized by thin and low mineralized, brittle enamel predisposing for erosion, abrasion and rapid disintegration.

The clinical pattern of ECC is rampant and characteristic (Milnes, 1996) and the maxillary incisors are often first involved. The initial appearance is white areas of demineralization on the surface enamel along the gingival line. The condition progresses so that the white spots become cavities that are discoloured to brown or black from stains in foods and drinks. If left untreated, the decay continues to such an extent that the crowns become weakened and fractured. This process may be so rapid that the parents perceive the teeth as defective from the moment of eruption. The mandibular incisors are normally protected by saliva from the submandibular/sublingual duct and the position of the tongue during feeding.

11.3 Prevention of ECC – main preventive strategies

Dental care is the most common unmet health care need of children (Mouradian, 2001). Thus, the promotion of oral health and preventive dental care are fundamental concepts in dentistry for children. In this context, the pediatric dentist has a very specific moral responsibility towards children and their parents as well as to society. Three main strategies have been described in preventive medicine (Rose, 1985). The *population strategy*, aimed for all individuals, whether diseased or not, was the dominant approach during the high caries era in the Nordic and many Western countries a few decades ago. Examples of such community-based activities are water fluoridation and dental education at oral well-baby evaluations. With decreasing prevalence and an increasing polarization of caries in the child populations, this strategy was called into question and the *high-risk strategy* emerged. The underlying thinking was that scarce resources should be concentrated on those individuals with the highest need. This approach requires simple and reliable test methods for the screening of high caries risk individuals if it is to be effective. A number of screening tests have been developed and evaluated for children and adolescents but concerns have been raised over the predictive ability of some of them (Hausen, 1997). Even when the past caries experience was used as a screening criterion, a great number of children were missed (false negatives) while other children not at risk were screened positive (false positives) and unnecessarily included in preventive programmes. A third, intermediary strategy is the *risk group strategy*, where efforts are targeted on selected groups in the community with a high caries level in an otherwise low caries population. Examples of the risk group approach can be found in North America with tailored activities directed to ethnic minority groups and Head Start Projects (Bruerd and Jones, 1996). It must however be strongly underlined that population strategies and high-risk strategies should not be regarded as alternatives but go hand in hand. The population strategies should aim at reducing the general level of risk factors in the population by general health promotion activities, while risk strategies should aim to control the disease in those individuals with clinical manifestations of a high disease activity.

11.4 Predictors of ECC and risk assessment

The object of identifying infants with an increased risk for a disease is to target and monitor the preventive treatment prior to clinical signs of onset. For an appropriate caries risk assessment, data obtained from the background factors and case history, clinical examination and bacterial tests must be put together to an individual profile (Newbrun, 1993). Although a great number of risk factors are strongly associated with ECC, this does not necessarily mean that they are causative or even useful as predictors for the disease. As discussed above, caries is multi-factorial in nature and the relative importance of the various etiologic factors may vary from one child to another. Thus, there is no single risk factor or risk indicator with enough predictive power to accurately select infants at risk. For example, studies of mutans streptococci as a single risk factor have indicated a high sensitivity but a poor specificity (Edelstein and Tinanoff, 1980). Therefore, combinations of clinical variables have been suggested to improve the process. Swedish investigators showed in a prospective study that predictors for caries development before 3.5 years of age were mutans streptococci colonization, immigrant background, frequent consumption of candy and sugar-containing beverages and mother's education (Grindefjord et al., 1996). The probability of caries development was 87% when all the variables were present at 1 year of age.

11.5 The preventive message – what do we communicate?

There are three principal ways to combat ECC, namely by

- community measures,
- professional measures
- home-care methods.

  Community based measures are mainly organized and provided by public health authorities, such as education programmes and water fluoridation, while the professional measures are conducted at the dental office. The home-based strategy involves the development and support of self-care habits such as oral hygiene routines, dietary and feeding habits as well as awareness and attitudes. The principles of caries prevention are well known and the basic message is listed in Table 11.2.

Table 11.2: The preventive message

- Do not put the pacifier or child's spoon in your mouth
- No sleeping with baby bottle, except with water in it
- Clean the teeth twice daily — after breakfast and before bedtime — with a soft baby toothbrush from the eruption of the very first tooth
- Use fluoridated toothpaste daily from the age of 12–18 months*)
- Limit the number of sweet drinks and snacks
- Perform regular examinations to identify plaque and decay — lift the lip

*) Comment of the editors: Dental Associations of many countries recommend this. However, the German Academy of Paediatrics (DAKJ) recommends fluoride supplements for the first three years of life which have been proven to effectively prevent dental caries and which are widely used in Germany. According to the DAKJ, fluoride toothpaste has not been tested systematically in infants and toddlers. Fluoride tooth paste is a cosmetic and does not consist of nutrients. Young children would swallow most of it regularly, which may not be desirable from a health point of view.

For a more thorough coverage of various preventive methods in early childhood, a textbook on preventive dentistry is advocated. Furthermore, a reference manual to current oral health policies within pediatric dentistry has recently been published and may serve as a guideline in this context (American Academy of Pediatric Dentistry, 1999). The cornerstones in caries prevention are fluoride, oral hygiene and diet. The common use of fluoride was ranked as the outstanding and single most important factor explaining the recent caries decline as judged by dental experts in a recent questionnaire (Bratthall et al., 1996). Here it can also be of interest to emphasize that the views on the anti-caries mechanisms of fluoride have undergone a paradigmatic shift during the recent decade. The systemic effect has been downgraded and the local upgraded. The current view is that fluoride has to be present in the plaque fluid during the caries challenge to slow down the dissolution of enamel and support the precipitation (remineralization) phase (ten Cate, 1999). After topical administration, calcium fluoride depots are formed on the tooth surface as a pH-controlled release system ready to act when needed (Øgaard et al., 1994). The local mode action has resulted in the fact that lozenges have replaced standard fluoride tablets and these are no longer recommended for children under the age of 3 years in Sweden (which is not the case in Germany; editors comment). Since the effective concentration of fluoride is directly dependent on the caries activity, children with ECC need frequent fluoride applications (Ismail, 1994). For young children with caries risk or with early signs of ECC, professional applications with fluoride varnish seem to be reasonably effective.

A novel approach in early caries prevention is to combat the cariogenic microorganisms with chemotherapeutic agents. The antibacterial measures can be directed either towards the caregivers or to their children. In the former case, the goal is to decrease or delay the transmission of mutans streptococci from mother to child. This can be achieved by cutting the main routes of transmission and by suppressing the levels of salivary mutans streptococci in highly-infected mothers (Tenovuo et al., 1992; Köhler and Andréen, 1994). Besides, pioneering studies have recently been presented in which the natural sugar alcohol xylitol was used to prevent mutans streptococci transmission and colonization by inhibiting the bacterial adhesion to enamel (Isokangas et al., 2000; Söderling et al., 2001). An example of the latter strategy is daily tooth brushing with a chlorhexidine gel, performed by the parents over a limited time period. (Twetman and Grindefjord, 1999).

11.6 Oral health education

Any preventive programme for ECC must provide support for and involve the participation of the parents or caregiver. Although the professionals can provide excellent care, in many countries without charges, the parents must be taught to take full responsibility for the oral health of their children. Secondly, dental education and preventive activities must start early, since the younger a person is, the easier it is to establish healthy habits. Furthermore, it has been shown that very young children with signs of caries tend to develop further caries in the primary dentition (O'Sullivan and Tinanoff, 1993; Grindefjord et al., 1995).

The goal of dental education is to improve the oral and feeding habits of parents or caregivers by increasing their knowledge about early childhood caries. This is mostly accomplished by cognitive-behavioural intervention. The key-person is without doubt the mother. In most cultures, she takes most responsibility for the care of the baby during the infant and toddler period. Moreover, several studies have shown that the mother's education status is inversely related to early caries prevalence and incidence (Grindefjord et al., 1995; Tang et al., 1997) and her beliefs do influence the likelihood of compliance. Thus, the oral health message should be *simple, consistent* and *evidence-based*. Although few studies have been designed to evaluate the effect of education on ECC, two contrasting views seem to dominate. One is that education alone is insufficient and ineffective to ensure a permanent change in health behaviour and relapses are inevitable (Kay and Locker, 1996; Reisine and Douglass, 1998). Others claim that education may have a positive and sustained impact on feeding patterns and tooth brushing (Bruerd and Jones, 1997; Harrison and White, 1997). In Sweden, systematic dental health counselling at child health centres (CHC) was introduced in the 1960s and the information was given on two occasions, when the child was 6−8 months and again at 18 months. Studies from the early 1970s reported positive effects of those activities with decreased caries levels in the 4-year-olds (Köhler and Holst, 1973; Holm, 1975).

However, a later evaluation stated that the dental information given at the CHCs was of negligible value with regards to the parent's general level of knowledge (Granath Kinnby, 1994). The vast majority understood the information but most of them did not learn anything new. This indicates that the information was not well adapted to the education level and social status of the recipients. It therefore seems of crucial importance to re-design the information to suit the prerequisites of the individual. Interestingly, the parents of caries-free children seemed to assimilate the information more actively. A key point may be that a continuous transfer of knowledge is essential for maintaining oral health. Experience from Scandinavia shows that the raising an almost caries-free generation does not mean that they, in turn, will automatically have caries-free children. The young parents are often unaware of the disease and do not consider the caries as a problem, and thus simply lack the knowledge about how to handle their children from a dental point of view.

Concluding the paragraphs above, dental health education is simply too important to be overlooked and extensive efforts are needed to review and improve the programmes. In this aspect, the collaboration with behavioural science may be needed in order to add knowledge and skills of dental personnel to change and modify patient behaviour (Schou, 2000). Although the efficiency still is somewhat uncertain, adapted oral health promotion programmes should be strongly recommended, implemented and provided for high-risk groups and high-risk communities. Information in early childhood gives the best results. Wherever possible, preventive oral health information should also be provided to expectant parents during prenatal education programmes.

11.7 How do we communicate the preventive message?

The information process includes absorbing, processing, interpreting and remembering information. Communication is an exchange of messages between a sender and a receiver. An effective information process calls for a two-way communication in which the parties are on balanced terms. In two-way communication the receiver is in a position to put questions and ask for explanations. At the same time, the sender is able to check whether the message is perceived correctly. The children are the third group in this communication process. The parents are instrumental in converting the accepted concept to a desired behaviour in their children by i.e. positive attitudes, good behaviour and reinforcement. Feedback is all the time of greatest importance for all parties involved. The parent's trust of and satisfaction with the caregiver is also of importance to the adherence of the message.

The choice of medium for the information is important. In general, personal influence and visual media seem to have a great advantage over printed material. The success of dental health education may further depend on psychosocial factors such as attitudes, self-esteem, immigrant status and level of social deprivation. As already mentioned, it is most important to individualize the information by inter-personal communication and tailor the advice to ethnic and age-specific conditions. This can be accomplished by enrolling lay-people in the process – *"from local people to local people"*. To educate and utilize dental health ambassadors with multicultural competence among various ethnic and social groups of the population may overcome many obstacles in the communication process and enhance the assimilation of the message. For obvious reasons, in most cases one-to-one educational settings are preferable to group counselling. The need for individualized information calls for an extended education in behavioural sciences among counselling dental personnel. Moreover, new media should be utilized and evaluated in order to stimulate and improve the information process.

11.8 The counselling situation

The primary objective in the counselling set-up is to convert pre-contemplating caregivers to contemplators. This means that those with no intention of changing unhealthy behaviour should be stimulated to consider making a change. This can be achieved by focusing the information on the benefits of being healthy rather than on a horror-scenario of the disease and its consequences. Information on the common barriers to change may be as important as the preventive message itself. Humour, pleasure and surprising people by saying or doing something "unexpected" may facilitate the information to be adopted. When the process of change is started, the support is merely focused on assisting the management of this process. A strategy for the counselling situation is suggested in Table 11.3.

Table 11.3: Suggested strategy for dental professionals in the individualised oral health information setting

- listen and understand, feed-back the child's personal risk
- define major problems
- discuss options to reduce risk, underline parent's personal responsibility for change
- suggest behaviour change strategies, offer a menu of options
- specify reachable and realistic intermediate and ultimate goals at implementation
- offer safe-for-teeth alternatives rather than prohibition
- encourage by active reinforcement of improvements, accept that lapses are natural, enhance optimism

In addition to the verbal information, model-learning activities may be effective in preventive dentistry. For example, "lift-the lip" technique means that parents and other caregivers are trained to regularly monitor the maxillary incisors and recognize early signs of plaque accumulation and early decay (Lee at al., 1994). The oral mucosa should also be evaluated since the presence of gingivitis may be an indicator of inadequate oral hygiene and increased caries risk. At the dentist's, plaque samples can be collected and evaluated with a simple chair-side technique (Dentocult®-Strip mutans, Helsinki, Finland). The number of mutans streptococci is displayed on a plastic strip that can be used as a diagnostic, didactic and motivating tool (Twetman et al., 1994). Other programmes are based on training the parents so that their children's teeth are adequately brushed. Such programmes have not only been implemented by society and local health authorities, but also by the industry. A number of successful oral hygiene teaching programmes in developing countries have been launched in collaboration with commercial companies. The marketing of sugar-free safe-for-teeth alternatives may also contribute to an increased awareness and a positive health behaviour.

Table 11.4: Organization of dental health activities during the first years of life within the Public Dental Service in Sweden

Time (age)	place	personnel	main objective
Pre-natal			
−3 months	clinic	maternal midwife	dental hygienist, oral hygiene during pregnancy, positive parenting
Post-natal			
6 months	centre	child health children's nurse	dental hygienist, importance of primary teeth, breast/bottle feeding, weaning tooth cleaning and use of fluoride
18 months	centre or dental clinic	child health	dental hygienist review parenting, oral inspection risk assessment, reinforcement intervention when needed
24−36 months	dental clinic	dentist	clinical examination, risk assessment individual recall based on risk, targeted preventive action

11.9 Collaborative programmes

ECC prevention is a public health goal. Thus, collaboration between dental, medical and social science and personnel is needed. A child at risk within one field is also often a risk patient for the other health care providers. It is important to utilize existing maternal and child services tied to the prenatal and well-baby visits. In 1973, the Act on Public Dental Service in Sweden made the county authorities responsible for providing a health-oriented dental care for everyone under the age of 19 years, free of charge. Although planned and implemented during the late 1960s, the programme still constitutes the core of the national oral health care. The basic organization during the first years of life is presented in Table 11.4. In recent years, some local alterations and modifications have been performed and the families can today freely choose between public and private clinics. At the beginning of the programme, dentists were conducting all the counselling and check-ups while today dental hygienists and specially trained nurses are the preventive front staff.

11.10 Summary

According to the United Nations' Convention on "The Rights of the Child", Articles 2 and 24, all children should have the same rights to health and medical service. Early childhood caries is a life-style disease with biological, behavioural and social determinants. Thus, ECC is a public health problem and health planners should give high priority to community-based comprehensive programmes with prenatal and postnatal education and motivation to prospecting parents as well as oral well-baby evaluations of their newly born children. A screening of all children at around 1–1½ years of age is an excellent opportunity for early detection of risk factors and risk indicators that may increase the possibilities for caries prevention. The risk evaluation should form the base for appropriate recommendations of preventive measures. The preventive care should equally be based on measures of the community, professional and self-care levels and the cornerstones are fluoride, oral hygiene and diet. Extended preventive programmes and activities should be organized and offered for risk groups (underprivileged, handicapped, medically compromised children) with an increased disease level compared to the norm. Behaviour science education of dental personnel should focus on improving the information and communication process and more applied research within this area is needed. Moreover, the various preventive interventions must be further developed and evaluated in prospective studies in terms of effectiveness and efficiency for infants and toddlers. This is an urgent task for health professionals and all societies with the ambition of providing good dental care for all young children.

11.11 References

[1] Alaluusua S, Renkonen OV: *Streptococcus mutans* establishment and dental caries experience in children from 2 to 4 years old. Scand J Dent Res 1983; 91: 453–457.
[2] American Academy of Pediatric Dentistry. Pediatr Dent 1999; 21 (Spec issue): 18–96.
[3] Barnes GP, Parker WA, Lyon TC, et al: Ethnicity, location, age and fluoridation factors in baby bottle tooth decay and caries prevalence of Head Start children. Public Health Rep 1992; 107: 167–172.
[4] Berkowitz RJ, Turner J, Green P: Maternal level of *Streptococcus mutans* and primary oral infection in infants. Arch Oral Biol 1981; 26: 147–149.
[5] Bratthall D, Hänsel-Petersson G, Sundberg H: Reasons for the caries decline: What do the experts believe? Eur J Oral Sci 1996; 104: 416–422.

[6] Bruerd B, Jones C: Preventing baby bottle tooth decay: eight year results. Public Health Rep 1996; 111: 63–65.

[7] ten Cate JM: Current concepts on the theories of the mechanism of action of fluoride. Acta Odontol Scand 1999; 57: 325–329.

[8] Caufield PW, Cutter GR, Dasanayake AP: Initial acquisition of mutans streptococci by infants: evidence for a discrete window of infectivity. J Dent Res 1993; 72: 37–45.

[9] Edelstein B, Tinanoff N: Screening preschool children for dental caries using a microbial test. Pediatr Dent 1980; 11: 129–132.

[10] Emanuelsson IR: Mutans streptococci – in families and on tooth sites. Studies on the distribution, acquisition and persistence using DNA fingerprinting. Swed Dent J. Suppl 2001; 148: 1–66.

[11] Flores G, Fuentes-Afflick E, Barbot O, et al: The health of latino children: urgent priorities, unanswered questions, and a research agenda. JAMA 2002; 288: 82–90.

[12] Grindefjord M, Dahllöf G, Modéer T: Caries development in children from 2.5 years of age: A longitudinal study. Caries Res 1995; 29: 449–454.

[13] Grindefjord M, Dahllöf G, Modéer T, et al: Prediction of dental caries development in 1-year-old children. Caries Res 1995; 29: 343–348.

[14] Grindefjord M, Dahllöf G, Nilsson B, et al: Stepwise prediction of dental caries in children up to 3.5 years of age. Caries Res 1996; 30: 256–266.

[15] Harrison R, White L: A community-based approach to infant and child oral health promotion in a British Columbia first nations community. Can J Community Dent 1997; 12: 7–14.

[16] Hausen H: Caries prediction – state of the art. Community Dent Oral Epidemiol 1997; 25: 87–96.

[17] Holm AK. Tandhälsa hos tre- till femåriga svenska barn (abstract). Umeå University Odontological Dissertations Abstracts. No 5. 1975.

[18] van Houte J: Role of microorganisms in caries etiology. J Dent Res 1994; 73: 672–681.

[19] Ismail AI: Fluoride supplements: current effectiveness, side effects, and recommendations. Community Dent Oral Epidemiol 22: 164–172, 1994

[20] Ismail AI: Prevention of early childhood caries. Community Dent Oral Epidemiol 1998;26 (Suppl 1): 49–61.

[21] Isokangas P, Söderling E, Pienihäkkinen K, et al: Occurrence of dental decay in children after maternal consumption of xylitol chewing gum, a follow-up from 0 to 5 years of age. L Dent Res 2000; 79: 1885–1889.

[22] Kay EJ, Locker D: Is dental health education effective? A systematic review of current evidence. Community Dent Oral Epidemiol 1996; 24: 231–235.

[23] Granath Kinnby C: On the value of dental health care information at child health centers. Lund University Odontological Dissertations, Malmö, 1994.

[24] Köhler B, Andréen I: Influence of caries-preventive measures in mothers on cariogenic bacteria and caries experience in their children. Arch Oral Biol 1994; 39: 907–911.

[25] Köhler B, Andréen I, Jonsson B: The earlier the colonization by mutans streptococci, the higher the caries prevalence at 4 years of age. Oral Immunol Microbiol 1988; 3: 14–17.

[26] Köhler L, Holst K: Dental health of four-year-old children. Acta Paediatr Scand 1973; 62: 269–278.

[27] Lee C, Rexaiamira N, Jeffcott E, et al: Teaching parents at WIC clinics to examine their high caries-risk babies. J Dent Child 1994; 61: 347–349.

[28] Milnes AR: Description and epidemiology of nursing caries. J Public Health Dent 1996; 56: 38–50.

[29] Mouradian WE: The face of a child: children's oral health and dental education. J Dent Educ 2001; 65: 821–831.

[30] Newbrun E: Problems in caries diagnosis. Int Dent J 1993; 43: 133–142.

[31] gaard, B Rölla G, Arends J: Professional topical fluoride applications – clinical efficiency and mechanism of action. Adv Dent Res 1994; 8: 190–201.

[32] O'Sullivan DM, Tinanoff N: Maxillary anterior caries associated with increased caries risk in other primary teeth. J Dent Res 1993; 72: 1577–1580.

[33] Reisine S, Douglass JM: Psychosocial and behavioural issues in early childhood caries. Community Dent oral Epidemiol 1998; 26 (Suppl 1): 32–44.

[34] Rose G: Sick individuals and sick populations. Int J Epidemiol 1985; 14: 32–38.

[35] Schou L: The relevance of behavioural science in dental practice. Int Dent J 2000; 50: 324–332.

[36] Seow WK: Biological mechanisms of early childhood caries. Community Dent Oral Epidemiol 1998; 26 (Suppl 1): 8–27.

[37] Söderling E, Isokangas P, Pienihäkkinen K, et al: Influence of maternal xylitol consumption on mother-child transmission of mutans streptococci: 6-year follow-up. Caries Res 2001; 35: 173–177.

[38] Tang JMW, Altman DS, Robertson DC, et al: Dental caries prevalence and treatment levels in Arizona preschool children. Public Health Rep 1997; 112: 65–75.

[39] Tinanoff N, Daley N, O'Sullivan D, et al: Failure of intense preventive efforts to arrest early childhood and rampant caries: three case reports. Pediatric Dentistry 1998; 21: 160–163.

[40] Tenovuo J, Hakkinen P, Paunio P, et al: Effects of chlorhexidine-gel treatments in mothers on the establishment of mutans streptococci in primary teeth and the development of dental caries in children. Caries Res 1992; 26: 275–280.

[41] Thorild I, Lindau-Jonson B, Twetman S: Prevalence of salivary mutans streptococci in mothers and in their preschool children. Int J Paediatr Dent 2002; 12: 2–7.

[42] Twetman S, Grindefjord M: Mutans streptococci suppression by chlorhexidine gel in toddlers. Am J Dent 1999; 12: 89–91.

[43] Twetman S, Ståhl B, Nederfors T: Use of the strip mutans test in assessment of caries risk in a group of preschool children. Int J Paediatr Dent 1994; 4: 245–250.

[44] Wendt L-K: On oral health in infants and toddlers. Swed Dent J 1995; Suppl 106.

12 Social backgrounds and communication strategies in family centred health promotion

Peter-Ernst Schnabel

12.1 Introduction

Family-oriented health promotion is still underdeveloped in Germany. This is not so much due to a general loss of function of the family in modern societies (Mitterauer & Sieder 1980) or to a crisis of the family (Lehr 1982), but depends mainly on the complex and widely unexplored health functions of families in our country, on the strict privacy which protects family life against influences from outside, and on the fact that social agencies may only intervene when a family is already in crisis and its members have proved beyond doubt that they cannot help themselves.

The combined result is that in nine out of ten cases, social or public health policy in Germany is dealing with crises, breakdowns and diseases and not with normality and health. A survey of family health promotion activities in Germany over the past ten to fifteen years (Schnabel 2000) suggests that in Germany most publicly organized and funded prevention or health promotion efforts occur much too late and use inappropriate means. The great majority of projects and programmes today concentrate on health promotion at work, that means mainly for middle-aged adults, for whom

- the probability of becoming chronically ill is increasing exponentially,
- the accumulated stress overload is high,
- the gap between the socio-/psychosomatic burdens and compensation possibilities is wide.

In contrast, family related health promotion includes the opportunity to intervene at a very early point in the development of the family system and its young members, when

- the burdens and the possibility of getting ill are low, and
- compensation is relatively simple, because
- children and their young parents still have relatively high physical and psychosocial health potential.

But one has to be careful. Families in a *risk society* like Germany (U. Beck (1986)) should not be overloaded with too many complex duties. And not all families are able to bear the same burdens, because they differ in terms of economic status, education, and the level of accessible social resources.

12.2 Disease – health – family. An ambivalent and relatively unknown triangle

Bearing the difficult situation of families in mind and their ambivalent functionality in modern societies, some studies in family health care stress that one can only identify and use the health potentials of families correctly by including the risks of family life; whether the knowledge is to be used for health promotion with normal families or families in risky situations. Badura and collaborators have worked this out clearly in the "Oldenburg Longitudinal Study" (Badura, Kaufholt, Lehmann, Pfaff, Schott & Walz 1987). They showed a positive correlation between the health gain of men recovering from cardiac infarction and their wives' probability of falling ill at the same time. This makes clear that every one who wants to mobilise the power and the special psycho-social potentials of the family in order to minimize risky health behaviour, should not do this without exact knowledge about those pathological and or health promoting effects in today's family life in the various social strata.

Today the majority of family studies still either concentrate on the healthy aspects and neglecting the pathological ones, or focus on the pathological effects of family life and overlook health potentials. The only exceptions seems to be a small number of very interesting and well-prepared case studies from the eighties (Wirsching & Stierlin 1982, Minuchin, Roseman & Baker 1983, Mattejat 1982) which tried and often succeeded to cope with psychiatric and psychosomatic diseases by influencing the ways of interaction and communication between family members. But as long as further studies of this quality are lacking, we can only construct models like the following (Fig. 12.1), only to maintain that kind of control over the development, influence and interaction of the pathological and healthy factors in the real family process, that family health promotion policy urgently needs.

This model, which tries to integrate the results of the last decade of illness- and health research is based on two interactive groups of dominating factors: family systemic factors (see the upper rows) and the individual factors (see the rows below), especially concerning the affairs of parents and children. Objective burdens on the family generate what Hurrelmann calls 'family-stress' (1990) and this can be passed right through to affect the health of individual family members.

The size of this effect depends on the interaction of many intervening social and economic factors, which can be classified as objective or actually effective ones. The

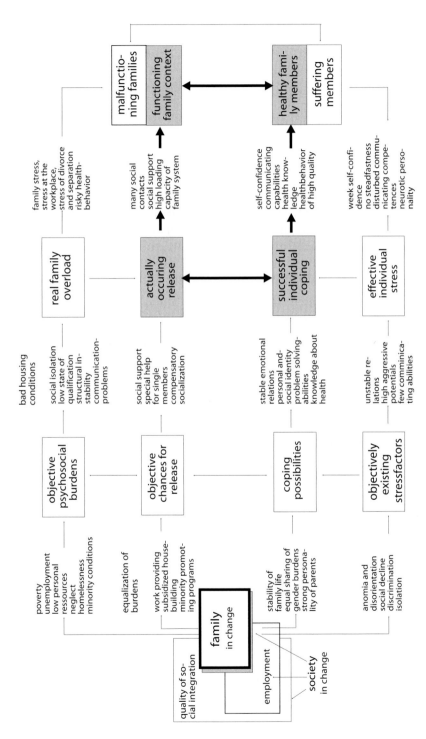

Fig. 1: Model of the process of family related salutogenesis

coping capacities of the family system and its individual members determine the susceptibility of the individuals or the family as a group. The message of the model is that children are more likely to develop in a healthy way within and by means of a functioning family context if the active burdens are low and the family system is fulfilling its many communication functions as socialization agent. (These include biological reproduction, upbringing and care, socialisation and social control, material and psycho-social regeneration.)

To understand the model, it has to be taken into consideration that the concept of family here is not restricted to the nuclear family constellation (two generations, two children), but includes all other forms of family life, including those with more than two generations in one household, single-parent families, or unmarried couples with several children, which altogether now represent about a third of German families. All play a role in social life, and must be considered in analysis and for psycho-social intervention as well, because each type of structure has typical burdens, can mobilize different potentials in different ways and therefore requires different health promoting instruments and strategies.

The parameters affecting individual and family health cannot be discussed in detail here, but they can be summarised as follows:

- The socio-economic status of families: It is still responsible for the diversification of individual and systemic health risks, as it was earlier for infectious diseases. Because of the special socio-psycho-somatic character, chronic diseases, which top the health and mortality statistics, seem to be much more influenced by education and professional qualification of family members, by love and affection, by social support and/or the amount of therapy and health promotion, a family can afford (Hurrelmann & Schnabel 1997).
- The socialization process: As a process of life-long learning, in which the family plays a primary and enduring part, it is responsible for the way in which successful families and their members solve problems caused by the management of diseases and health protection (Hurrelmann 2000). In the course of socialization, skills of adaptation, self-determination, problem solving and so on are developed which are crucial if individuals and family groups are to cope with stress potentials of every day life in a less self-destructive manner.
- Verbal and nonverbal communication: This plays an important role in the life-long process of personality formation and the acquisition of life skills. Communication makes it possible for individuals to learn from each other and define their social position by exchanging socio-emotional, expressive and rational messages (Habermas 1981). Social systems such as families communicate too, in order to differentiate themselves from other systems or to open themselves to influences from outside, and they are forced to communicate both internally and externally to mobilize the potential of members and the family system as a whole against threats to health and disruption.

- The family cycle: It is nearly impossible, to recognize family related health risks and to cope with them adequately, if you do not realize the position of the family in what is called the family cycle (Textor 1984). Because some of these positions − in the mean time five rather important ones have been identified by biographical research − are characterized by a typical constellation of burdens, potentials, attainable help and stress, they affect family health status in many ways. Family health promotion could probably be improved substantially if experts were able to use these typically varying health potentials or health motifs, as identified by Enger & Grunow (1987) in a very interesting study in the 1980s.

We are now able to define health as the complex ability to organize and maintain a healthy life process by developing and exercising skills of communication; a process in which family plays a fundamental, life-long role. This ability includes the communication about diseases and other handicaps, but by no means should be identified with it. The process of its acquisition can be passed through more satisfyingly by the individual and more successfully by the family system, if the stages of development are completed one after another, as well as and in accordance with the physical and psychic development of family members and the changing needs of family life. Because of this, family oriented health promotion should do everything to support families in effectively playing their central and increasingly difficult role as socialization agencies.

12.3 Family oriented health promotion − the international situation

Well-documented projects show that the quality of publicly-accepted ideas or models about the family's influence on health predetermine the ways by which health promotion is realized internationally − whether in communities, schools, companies or in the family setting. Besides this, it has to realized in accordance with the Jakarta Declaration on Health Promotion into the 21st Century (WHO 1997), that the enduring success of interventions correlates positively with the analytical and conceptional quality of programmes and with the strategic ability of promotion experts to meet the real needs of population.

In spite of this, the great majority of programmes and family health promotion projects all over the world concentrate on families with high risks and on family members recuperating from diseases, psychiatric lesions and other handicaps. In most cases parent-child-relations are used to secure children's compliance or the family serves as therapeutic medium to cure individuals by improving the styles of internal communication and the quality of family relations. Most of these activities are purely reactive, and are characterized by their dependency on experts and their focus on the elimination of defects and deficits by means of pedagogic deterrence.

In contrast, only a few initiatives concentrate on the health of normal families in a threatening world and about families in different stages of development. It takes a long time to find out German programmes or projects which would stand comparison with American programmes like "Child and Adolescent Trial for Cardiovascular Health" (CATCH) (Edmundson et al. 1996), like the "SUPER STARS" programme on promoting health protection, especially psychosocial factors by means of the family (Emshoff et al. 1996) or the "Family First Program" against child abuse and neglect (Shuerman, Rzepnicki & Littell 1994), especially regarding the strategic complexity or organizational and instrumental inputs. And one would have a hard time looking in Europe for seventy model projects, such as those evaluated by the "Harvard Family Research Project" (1995) some years ago. All together there are good reasons to argue for changes to existing strategies and to plead for a policy of family empowerment, in order to push forward family health promotion more successfully.

12.4 Suggestions for a communications-centred strategy for family related health promotion

I would like to propose the development and realization of a family related policy for health promotion which would improve efficiency by drawing strategic consequences from the following insights:

The instruments by which health promotion in general has been promoted in recent decades bring about quite different results, depending on the setting and the specific objectives for setting them in action

The permanency of promotion effects varies according with the degree by which promotion experts succeed in combining more than one setting and different intervention methods to fit as closely as possible to the needs of family members

The persistency of effects depends on the degree to which the instruments chosen correspond to the typical problems taking place during family life cycle as well as to the changing risks and health potentials.

The strategy itself should be divided into five modules (Fig. 12.2).

Each module can be implemented separately, but the strategy can and should also be taken as a problem oriented, family related promotion policy covering the complete family cycle and the life span of family members. Experts who are charged with the planning and realization of single parts as well as with the policy as a whole, are well advised to take into account three very important aspects:

- The changing problem and support history of families,
- The adequacy of targets, instruments and settings and
- The strategic fit of the different instruments of intervention to the problems that have to be solved.

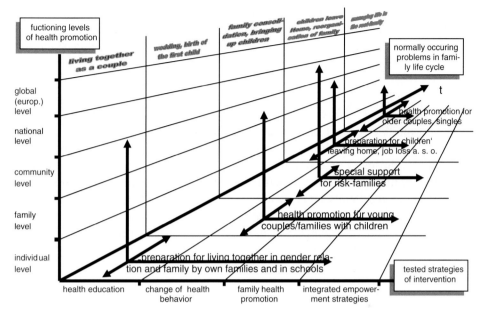

Fig. 12.2: Dimensions and modules of an integrated strategy of family health promotion

This change of procedure should be seen as a necessary investment in the future of family health promotion, because concentrating on certain particular professional interests has proven rather ineffective in the past. The strategy presented here not only offers more options for scientific research and practical intervention. Additionally the suggestion is made here, to add another four modules to the classic one, which neglects normal family life, strictly concentrates on problem families and diseases and as such still represents the majority of recent activities in Germany.

12.4.1 First module

The first module aims at the improvement of communication abilities, to help young people to cope with the problems of child-parent and gender relations and with the establishment of their own partnerships and functioning families. It starts at school and draws much of its strength from the cooperation with parents, adequate regional institutions and with peer-groups in their special activities. From the very few programmes and projects of this type, we know that the effective instruments include coeducative project teaching, problem oriented working groups of pupils, teachers and parents as well as regional cooperative programmes, dealing with the analysis and the improvement of adolescent and adolescent-adult relations in everyday life (Hildebrandt 1987). Families, parents, teachers, social workers and other experts are advised not to confront adolescents with draconian prohibitions or with behaviour expectations, that must appear dishonest to them and/or push them into conflicts with their peers (Franzkowiak 1993). Good experience has been made however, if parents or external experts manage to combine health targets with the typical wants of adolescents for originality, identity, mobility, fitness, attractiveness and adventure (Hurrelmann 2000).

12.4.2 Second module

The second module focuses on mastering problems with family foundation, especially with the birth of children and the many changes this brings in the sexual, emotional, psychosocial or economical aspects of gender relations. In connection with this, initiatives proved to be useful which tried to combine instruments of behaviour training and family advice with a stable, cheap and freely accessible supply of services, like those found in American Health Centres (Otto & Flösser 1992). In Germany they could be organized in part by adult colleges, institutions of family education or special self-help initiatives.

12.4.3 Third module

The third module concentrates on special support strategies for families in difficult situations or for risk families. Risk families have to fight very hard for the consolidation of the family system, and a pleasant social and economic outcome; that means for the fulfilment of even basic social needs. This is true for families with a number of children, for families with small incomes and children, for step families with more than two children, for single-parent families, and the support is needed even more by families which combine several psychosocial risks, like poor unmarried couples with several children in changing conditions, or no-income single-parent families, etc. (Hurrelmann & Schnabel 1997).

12.4.4 Fourth module

In the fourth module most of the initiatives are directed towards the improvement of coping and communication skills, which can help with reorganisation problems that can arise when children leave home, when mothers go back to work, or when husbands have to prepare for every day life as pensioners. Research has shown that in this phase of family life, existing and/or newly-developed health motives and leisure time can play an important role in the rebuilding of the somatic and psychosocial potentials which have been exhausted during the family consolidation phases. It can also be helpful to engage in special therapies and health promotion initiatives both at the individual and family or communal levels. But we have to register too that especially in Germany tried and tested instruments and strategies of this kind are still lacking, not to mention programmes that take special care of this family situation.

12.4.5 Fifth module

The fifth module, finally, should care for lonely and socially-isolated couples and individuals, with information events, training courses, working groups, or excursions. These initiatives should be intellectually and physiologically stimulating. They should be designed and implemented as integral parts of programmes for the establishment of comprehensive systems of residential outpatient care. The main purpose of such programmes is to maintain physical and intellectual independence of the elderly by enabling them to stay active for as long as possible. Therefore represent a much more humane alternative to the strategy of separation and hospitalisation that is dominant in Germany.

It is quite clear, that neither one of these modules nor the strategy as a whole will have a chance unless at least the first three of the following framework conditions are also implemented:

- Finding and maintaining the personnel, funds, time and curricular space within families, schools and services, which is necessary to set these alternative policies and the many related steps into motion,
- Convincing the management of business companies, administrations and other institutions which are busy organizing every-day life, to invest much more energy and resources into the health and future of their personnel, clients and customers,
- Improving the ability and willingness of health boards or other institutions of good-standing to engage in the planning, coordination and/or evaluation of family related and other health promoting activities,
- Establishing in law the claim to a publicly funded policy of health promotion as an equivalent principle of public welfare,
- And finally, in the distant future, the establishment of a constitutional right to grow up in health in a pleasant and compatible social and material environment.

12.5 Conclusion

Family oriented health promotion, understood as an integrated and enduring strategy, aimed at improving and/or stabilising family systems and strengthening the health potential of the family members, has not only to be seen as an investment in the future of society's health. Although it is still underestimated by scientists, politicians, the lay public, after more intervention studies and programmes, it could prove to be one of the most effective and worthwhile measures against the spread of the well known chronic diseases, which will continue to dominate the health situation of modern societies for the foreseeable future.

12.6 References

[1] Badura B., Kaufholt G., Lehmann H., Pfaff H., Schott T. & Walz W. (1987). Leben mit dem Herzinfarkt. Eine sozialepidemiologische Studie. Berlin: Springer.

[2] Beck U. (1986). Risikogesellschaft. Der Weg in eine andere Moderne. Frankfurt a. M.: Suhrkamp.

[3] Edmundson E. et al. (1996). The Effects of the Child and Adolescent Trial for Cardiovascular Health Intervention on Psychosocial Determinants of Cardiovascular Disease Risk Behavior among Thrird-Grade Students. American Journal of Health Promotion 10 (3), 217–225.

[4] Emshoff J. et al. (1996). Findings from SUPER Stars; A Health Promotion Program for Families to E Multiple Protective Factors. Journal of Adolescent Research 11 (1), 68–96.

[5] Engfer R. & Grunow D. (1987). Gesundheitsbezogenes Alltagshandeln im Lebenslauf. Bielefeld: B. Kleine Verlag.

[6] Habermas J. (1981). Theorie des kommunikativen Handelns. Frankfurt a. M.: Suhrkamp.

[7] Havard Family Research Project (1995). Raising our Future. Families, Schools and Communities Together. Cambridge/Mass.: Havard School of Education.

[8] Hurrelmann K. (1990). Familienstress Schulstress, Freizeitstress. Gesundheitsförderung für Kinder und Jugendliche. Weinheim: Beltz.

[9] Hurrelmann K. (1991). Sozialisation und Gesundheit. Somatische, psychische und soziale Risikofaktoren im Lebenslauf. Weinheim & Munich: Juventa.

[10] Hurrelmann K. (2000). Gesundheitssoziologie. Eine Einführung in sozialwissenschaftliche Theorien von Krankheitsprävention und Gesundheitsförderung. Weinheim & Munich: Juventa.

[11] Lehr U. (1982). Familie in der Krise. Plädoyer für mehr Partnerschaft in Ehe, Familie und Beruf. Munich: Olzog.

[12] Lobnig H. u. a. (Ed.) (1997). Gesundheitsförderung in Settings: Gemeinde, Betrieb, Schule. Krankenhaus – eine östreichische Forschungsbillanz. Vienna: Facultas.

[13] Mattejat F. (1985). Familie und psychische Störungen. Stuttgart: Enke.

[14] Mitterauer M. (1980). Funktionsverlust der Familie ? In: M. Mitterauer & R. Sieder (Hrsg.) Vom Patriarchat zur Partnerschaft. Munich: Pieper, 92–113.

[15] Minuchin A., Rosman B. & Baker L. (1983). Psychosomatische Krankheiten in der Familie. Stuttgart: Klett Cotta.

[16] Mitscherlich A. (1974). Krankheit und Konflikt. Frankfurt a. M.: Suhrkamp.

[17] Pelikan J. M., Demmer H. & Hurrelmann K. (1993). Gesundheitsförderung durch Organisationsentwicklung. Konzepte, Strategien und Projekte für Betriebe, Krankenhäuser und Schulen. Weinheim & Munich: Juventa.

[18] Schnabel P.-E. (1988): Krankheit und Sozialisation. Vergesellschaftung als pathogener Prozess. Opladen: Westdeutscher Verlag.

[19] Schnabel P.-E. (2000). Familie und Gesundheit. Bedingungen , Möglichkeiten und Konzepte der Gesundheitsförderung. Weinheim & Munich: Juventa (in print).

[20] Schuerman J. R., Rzepnicki T. L. & Littell J. H. (1994). Putting Families First. An Experiment in Family Preservation. New York: de Gruyter.

[21] Textor M. R. (1984). Erziehung im Familienzyklus. In: M. R. Textor (Hrsg.). Die Familie. Frankfurt a. M.: Haag & Herchen, 65–90.

[22] Wirsching M. Stierlin H. (1982). Krankheit und Familie. Konzepte – Forschungsergebnisse – Therapie. Stuttgart: Klett Cotta.

[23] World Health Organisation (WHO) (ed.) (1997). The Jakarta Declaration on Health Promotion into the 21st Century. Jakarta/Indonesia.

12.7 Discussion

Dr. Bergmann:
Now I have a question: you wanted to tell us something about a change of policy to improve our communication strategies for the sociallyisolated. Can you tell us something about this?

Prof. Schnabel:
Yes. The last module − yes. Several things on many layers, you have to start with one, it would to get the free-room in schools and families and in other institutions in a region to improve the interest for health. All people have to do with illness, and look for their cure and care, but it would not be enough for their health and therefore you need free-room in the curricula of schools, in lifestyles of families, and for instance with the companies around where the people work, and there you have to install new ideas of health promotion. This is the first, the second is convincing the management of enterprises in a region, improving the capability and readiness of health boards in the same region, and other institutions, and establishing for people a claim to a socially organized and publicly funded prevention policy, and placing it beside the idea of subsidiarity as a second equivalent principle of state action.

Prof. Tietze (Chair):
Further questions? So I would like to ask a question: I refer to your very first slide, and you presented a quite complex model with many arrows. First question is: are these arrows meant in a sense of a causal relationship? Secondly: how much is the whole complex system really data-based? I mean, do we have knowledge enough, can we estimate effects which are growing from one source of influence to the next one? So I think it is important to see how all the things are inter-connected in order to plan appropriate interventions. So my question is how much is it really data-based, secondly what are the final criteria, what does it actually mean and how do you measure health of family members? Because health obviously is a very complex construct. I assume this is a kind of model which is based on correlation studies − do we have enough evidence, say, to plan interventions at a certain point, what would the effects of those interventions really be like? Because I think to have this technology in mind is a prerequisite for planning public strategies.

Prof. Schnabel:
No, this model is not data-based in the sense that you have data for each step connecting it with the next one. You have research between coping possibilities and successful individual coping. You have research between family and change and objectively existing stress factors, you have research between real family overload and actual relief, but not for the whole model. This is a difficult situation for health promotion, and therefore I am arguing that as long as you have no data bases for

these complex models you have to combine these single findings by a very plausible theoretical model. And the basis of my theoretical model are two groups of factors: a family life cycle and the socialization process in the family. This is very well described in research, pedagogical and psychological research.

Prof. Tietze (Chair):
May I add a question: When you say this is not that much data-based and we do not have comprehensive data-based models, how can we justify planning public strategies and asking for public money? Because I think to implement strategies in the way you have it in mind, we need to justify possible effects, otherwise I do not see how we can convince tax-payers in the end to invest in public health strategies.

Prof. Schnabel:
(What should I answer? There are more questions to this?) The problem is that no one, no institution and no single person would finance a project which can prove this model as a whole. It must be a longitudinal study, which controls longer processes of life, very complex processes. So if you insist on a data-based model in this way, you couldn't get active as a health promoter, but I think nothing speaks against a strategy of working with family life on the basis of this model, and I found examples for this in America. There are some projects in risk-factor prevention in working with families in ghettoes all connected in a Harvard family research project, they evaluated about seventy projects which work on the basis of such complex models and are very successful in the long run, but some of these models took 20 years to get a provable outcome.

Prof. Tietze (Chair):
Okay. A last question from the audience? Okay, so thank you very much for your contribution.

Index